AUTISM RECIPE
Using Trust and Joy to Take Control of Wellness

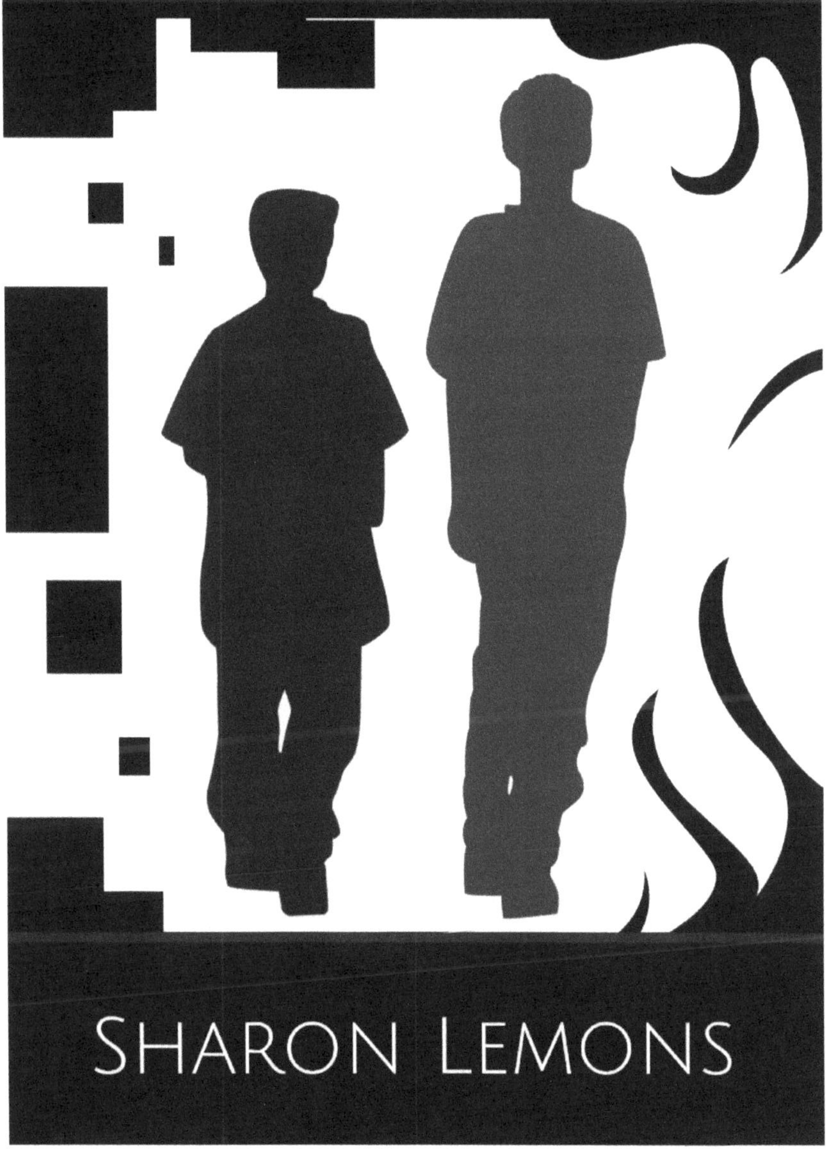

SHARON LEMONS

Copyright © 2023 by Sharon Lemons

All rights reserved. This book or any portion thereof may not be reproduced or used in any manner whatsoever without the express written permission of the publisher except for the use of brief quotations in a book review.

Printed in the United States of America

First Printing, 2023

ISBN 979-8-9888989-1-7

Lemons Nutrition

www.AutismRecipe.com

Acknowledgments

Over the years, many people have supported our journey and inspired us. While there are too many to list, I want to acknowledge some of the most influential.

Educators: Beth Beason, Robin Crosthwaite, Lainey Bauer, Charlene McClaren, Carol Dunham, Annette Nutter, Luke Schmidt, Vonda Brown (The Vonda Factor), David Forbus, Brenda Ornelas, Coach Hutton. I also want to mention that, frequently, teachers and school support staff were instrumental. I often relied on bus drivers to set the mood for the day or help transition the boys to a better mood after they left the school before reaching home. I was always grateful for any support, from any and all sources.

Beta Readers: I cannot begin to express my gratitude to those who read part or all of the book before we started editing: Bill Still, Lee Shelly Wallace, Paula Halbach, Jennifer Meyer, Kari Moore, Annette Nutter, Amanda Towns, Terry Flory, Joe McDaniel, Joan Medlin, Cindi Mitchell. Whether you read a little or a lot and suggested a lot of edits or none or affirmed you thought the book would benefit others, your time has meant the world to me!

My Editor: Karen, you are my cousin by birth and my very dear friend by choice. To say this book improved exponentially with your help is a MAJOR understatement. I am thankful for your editing skills and willingness to honestly share your opinions on what needed to be changed. I love you, my dear cousin and editor.

My Family: Obviously, this book would not have happened without our shared journey through autism. I want to especially thank you for being willing to allow our stories to be told, but also for the day-to-day support you all provide. What may not come across in the book is how spoiled I am by all of you. James, Richard, and Jason, you truly do more taking care of me than I do taking care of you these days. Justin, while you now live in another state, your support has been just as valuable as the support of your Dad and brothers. I truly appreciate your emotional support. I can't imagine navigating this journey without all of you. I love you all.

Graphic Artist: Richard, your talent amazes me! I am forever grateful for you and all the time you have spent making my ideas come to life in graphic form. Your contribution to this book has been immense!

Dedication

This book is dedicated to my family. Obviously, I would not have learned as much about autism without Richard and Jason, but everyone has always pulled together with a concerted effort to do the very best we could as a synchronized unit.

Richard, you brought us into the journey and left us amazed and inspired from the very beginning, whether it was sounding like a little professor when you talked or amazing everyone with your knowledge of dinosaurs and eventually completing college. We hold your accomplishments in high esteem.

Jason, you keep this family running, but your organization and drive to keep everything running smoothly extends not only to us, your immediate family, but also to the dedication and work you willingly undertook to help take care of your grandmothers. We know your employer appreciates your selfless commitment to purpose. You are a treasure.

Justin, nobody understands how much this journey affects a family more than you. Many has been the time we needed you to be an adult before you reached adulthood. We appreciate you and your love of our family more than can be put into words. I hope someday you choose to tell your side of the story. I know you could teach us all some of the nuances that can only be seen from a sibling's perspective.

James, you are my rock and my strength. You have put up with every crazy idea I have come up with and even managed to help me see the logic that I was willing to overlook in my zest to provide our boys with all the tools they need to be successful, healthy, and happy. I would not have wanted to have anyone else as my coadventurer on this quest.

Foreword

I still remember the first day I met Sharon Lemons. I was working in my University Feeding Clinic and, one day, this lady showed up with our New Eval. Turned out she was a dietitian, of all things. She was referring this little guy on her caseload for feeding therapy, and she even came along for the assessment. There wasn't an occupational therapist available in our state's Early Childhood Intervention program and this dietitian was determined to get the right resources for the families she served. Apparently knew a thing or two about feeding therapy, too. I really enjoyed having her there to provide her perspective along with the child's parents, and my students got to learn more about professional collaboration. After that she brought us kiddo after kiddo. She worked with the families in their homes encouraging carryover and working on *what* to feed these little ones. We had an amazing success rate that year. I wish I could take credit, but it was Sharon. I learned later she had walked this road personally with two of her own sons. She knew what it felt like not to be able to feed your own child. She knew what it felt like to scramble and scrounge to find *something* her sons would eat. She knew the results of therapists using M&Ms as behavioral reinforcers and having to pay tens of thousands of dollars for dental rehabilitation. She had been the scared, discouraged mom being told to expect the worst. *And she wasn't having it!*

How do you help a child with Autism Spectrum Disorder eat healthy foods? It seems impossible some days. And it did for Sharon, too. But out of all her personal and professional experiences comes a wealth of information on how to do just that, using trust and joy to take control of wellness instead of settling for just anything and hoping for the best.

Follow her journey and learn from one of the best pediatric feeding specialists I know!

Jennifer Meyer, MA, CCC-SLP

Table of Contents

Introduction 11
Chapter One 14
    Crash Course in Autism 14
    People-First 24
Chapter Two 29
    Hopes and Dreams 29
    The Challenge 37
    Different Perspectives 41
    Having a Hard Time 43
Chapter Three 48
    Trust and Joy 48
    The Essential Ingredient 51
    The Apple Test 56
    Behavior is Communication 62
    Dealing with Other People's Expectations 68
    Walking a Tight Rope 72
    Pressure-Free Zone at Mealtime 74
Chapter Four 85
    Meal Planning 85
    Starting Point 87
    Teaching Opportunities 90
    Taming the Snack Monster 93
    Lemons Food Project to the Rescue! 95
    Be Positive! 98
    Lemons Family Dinner Ground Rules 99
    Our Journey 101
    Making it Work for the Long Term 104
    A Word about Sweets and Serving Sizes 107
    Our Planning Process 108
    Mealtime Management 119
    Making it Work for You 120
    The Starting Point 122
    Adding New Foods 124
    Increasing Acceptance 125
    Creating Your Own Framework 127
    Contingency Meals 131

Food Prep and Kitchen Skills 132
Eating Away from Home 134
Finishing Up 137
Chapter Five 143
    Sensory Explorations 143
    Looking for Triggers 150
    Feeding Therapy 153
    Sensory Spectrum 156
    Sounds of Foods 162
    Texture of Food 164
    Aromas of Foods 167
    Tasting Foods 170
    Prepare for Change 172
Chapter Six 174
    Using Stories to Expand Food Selections 174
    Formulating a Story Plan 176
    Appropriate Stories 181
    Too Old for Stories? 182
    Next Steps 183
    Contingency Plans 185
    My First Food Story 189
Chapter Seven 195
    Special Diets 195
    Allergies 196
    Second Visit 197
    Testing the Corn Theory 200
    Autism Diet 201
    A Word about Supplements 206
    Isolation 207
    Spending Time with Friends 209

Chapter Eight ... 211
    You Don't Have to Be Perfect ... 211
    Change the Narrative! ... 214
    Therapy-Free Meals ... 215
    Changing Circumstances ... 216
    Building in Some Unpredictability ... 218
    Health Issues ... 219
    Methods for Dealing with an Unfamiliar Food ... 221
    Crisis ... 223
Chapter Nine ... 226
    Medical Wellness ... 226
    Keeping Up with Scheduled Maintenance ... 229
    Health Screening Recommendations ... 231
    Medications ... 235
    Other Skills Needed ... 236
    Activity ... 239
    Self-care ... 243
Chapter Ten ... 245
    Stepping out into the World ... 245
    Ordering Food ... 246
    Balancing Nutrition While Eating Out ... 248
    Frugal Eating ... 251
    Conquering the Grocery Store ... 252
    Becoming Mobile ... 254
    Entering the Workforce ... 259
    Challenges along the Way ... 263
Conclusion ... 268
    Take Home Messages ... 268
References ... 274
Appendix ... 285

Introduction

"He will never hold a pencil, much less write his name." The year was 1988, and the bleak pronouncement sent me into a combination of disbelief, denial, and anger. As the words of the occupational therapist cut through me like a knife, I began planning ways in my head to conquer whatever diagnosis she thought had a grip on my almost five-year-old son. She insisted Richard's fine motor skills were so bad he would never gain full use of his hands. As soon as we returned home, I pulled out the Pac-Man game to work on his fine motor skills. Then, when he could beat the game that evening, I pulled out the Etch a Sketch. Within the week, he had drawn dinosaurs on the Etch A Sketch, beaten Pac-Man quicker than I could, and written his name. He conquered these tasks before we returned for the follow-up assessment a few weeks later. When he graduated from the Art Institute with an associate degree in graphic arts, twenty-five years later, I sent that occupational therapy group an invitation to the ceremony without explaining or commenting to the practice that their therapist did not believe my son would ever hold a pencil.

Richard is not my only son with autism, and while this book is not a biography, it will include many stories of our experiences as parents of two children with autism. I want to share with you, dear reader, some of our journeys to give you a better perspective on how my conclusions formed and how I came to espouse some philosophies on autism. The stories I share are mainly from both my perspective as a parent and as a professional. Still others are about people in our lives who have traits of autism, but do not have a diagnosis. Generally, most people can identify some traits of autism in themselves when presented with a list of characteristics. I fall into that category, as I also have traits of autism, but no diagnosis. So, as I write this book, I draw on my experiences as a parent, my personal characteristics and those of others I know, as well as how we have all addressed our challenges. Out of respect for privacy, I do not always identify the people in my stories, as not everyone I talk about has a diagnosis nor wants to be named in a book; however, they do have these traits. All these experiences add to the possible strategies others might want to try when overcoming their own hurdles. To that end, the strategies I discuss here have value and diverse perspectives that anyone can use. I have undertaken this book in hopes that you, my readers, will find compassion, help, and joy as you create your own recipe for navigating your autism adventures.

Chapter One

Crash Course in Autism

Although it feels as if I have spent my entire life working with autism, it has really just been my adult life. On the day my oldest son, Richard, turned five, our world spun out of orbit as a psychologist, who needed some serious coaching in bedside manner, repeated the words the occupational therapist had first said a few weeks before. "Your son will never hold a pencil, let alone write his name." He stated it as bluntly as if he had just said my son had a cold. I stared at him in shock, his words a lightning bolt that shattered my heart. I was a twenty-eight-year-old mom looking forward to celebrating my child's birthday later that day. My youngest son, Jason, was three years old and exhibited many of the same traits as Richard, filling my heart with fear. It was more than my mind could fully absorb in one day.

I struggled to focus as the doctor continued, delivering Richard's vague diagnosis of PDD-NOS (Pervasive Developmental Disorder – Not Otherwise Specified), or as many parents call it now, "Pediatrician Did not Decide." His words were an ominously rolling thunderclap that would intensify to a resounding BOOM when my second son turned five years old, and the word autism was spoken. However, on that day Richard received his PDD-NOS diagnosis, the psychologist told us he wasn't precisely autistic, but wasn't ADD either. The silver lining was that we were told he would most likely have to work so hard to fit in, that by the time he was ten, he probably would be at or above his age level.

Two years later when our middle son, Jason, turned five, he also had a psychology appointment, and my fears were confirmed. The doctor diagnosed him with autism. During this appointment, I told the doctor about Richard, as well, since the boys had very similar behaviors. He spent extra time to explain to us that, no, Richard would *not* be miraculously fine by age ten, as the earlier psychologist had told us, and that we needed to prepare for a long "row to hoe." I held my one-week-old son and tried to absorb this news. The doctor looked at me and said, "Hand me the baby." I handed Justin over, and after a few moments of evaluation, he assured me he did not see any signs of autism in the baby. Then, he continued reviewing Richard's traits.

We discussed how on the day of Richard's earliest fine motor evaluation with the occupational therapist back in 1988, we were not yet concerned about Jason because his progress through various developmental milestones was similar to Richard's. The occupational therapist, however, had pointed out then that the fine motor skills causing her concern with Richard should have been developed by the age of two years old. When I told her our three-year-old, Jason, was not doing those specific things either, she had said, "You may have two on your hands."

I told the doctor how neither of the boys had much functional language. Richard could say hundreds of words because early on, when we became concerned about a lack of language, I would say words to him over and over until he repeated them, but he had no idea what they meant. Jason would say only Mama between screaming, blood-curdling cries when he wanted my attention. The psychologist listened attentively as I relayed all of this and encouraged me to call him if I "became concerned." The irony of those words! Thus began my autism adventures and education in earnest.

So let me explain that last qualifier, "in earnest." Previously, I had tried to learn everything I could to be a better parent, believing we were somehow doing something wrong. After the diagnosis, I read everything I could get my hands on and attended every training opportunity I could afford. Most of the information I found was helpful parenting advice. The data I received about diet modifications I'll call costly, and I'll address my thoughts on diets for autism in a separate chapter. There always seemed to be someone with "the answer." Many of these treatments are no longer around. We lived a comfortable life, financially speaking, at this point. That said, we did not have disposable income to support many of the treatments being encouraged, yet we earned too much to qualify for aid. Frankly, I am glad we missed out on treatments we could not afford. Some proved to have risks I would not have wanted to take, while other costly treatments later proved ineffective or simply disappeared.

After discussing things with the psychologist who diagnosed Jason, I dove even deeper into learning about autism. My husband once said, "You know so much more about autism than me." I answered, "Well, honey, you would have to quit your job to read and research about forty hours a week." It seemed that my knowledge increased every time there was a new challenge. I believe this is not an unusual parent response. I'm sure many parents reading this book have experienced the same thing. For the most part, I think parents do the best they can with the information they have at the time. I also believe the best therapist for these children is the parent, unless circumstances prevent them from it. Let me clarify that statement. I am not saying parents need to quit their jobs and do nothing but perform therapy for their children. I am also not saying that licensed therapists cannot play a significant role. I *am* saying that when teaching necessary day-to-day skills, every family has different dynamics. Nobody, except the parents, will teach a child to do every chore and handle every social skill the exact way it is typically done within your family. Heck, there are times I teach the boys how to do a task, then my husband turns around and asks them where they learned to do that? He then reteaches the tasks the way *he* prefers to do the task. We probably have learned more often which habits we have that annoy the other because we tried to untrain the boys in a pattern taught by the other one than from any other way.

Through our various trial and error experiences, I continued to sponge up all the information on autism I could find. I was willing to do whatever I could to enrich the experience of their lives. I am sure those of you reading this feel the same. When our boys received their diagnoses in 1988, and 1990, the officially accepted incidence of autism was reported to be four in 10,000.

While many people felt we were overly willing to try anything; others became frustrated because we did not try their latest suggestion. The internet was not available at that time, so my information came from reading a plethora of books and research studies, going to presentations on parenting, talking to educators, and making expensive long-distance phone calls. Many of the books that were available were written either by parents or by professionals that had something to sell. I learned through discussions with professionals I trusted to look closely at the source of information. They each had researchers they trusted and those they did not. I learned to look closely for the motives of those writing books and research papers. I also watched them closely at conferences. If they were wearing really expensive clothes and driving high end cars, I steered clear. Our philosophy was to do everything we could to help the boys within reason. Sometimes that "within reason" exception frustrated others. We did not give the strategies and those promoting them carte blanche with our financial resources.

An example of something we tried that was costly and

unsuccessful was a university program to determine what supplements might be beneficial. Additionally, there were a few individual supplements we tried. Here is how it worked out: The university program turned out to be a bust. After three months of giving the boys a concoction of pudding and supplements faithfully every day, we saw no benefit from the supplements. Worse yet, *both* wet the bed every single day for those three months. I finally gave up and ceremoniously threw all the supplements in the trash. I felt entitled to that show of emotion after washing all those sheets.

The individual supplements we tried in addition to those of the university program were a mixed bag of semi-success and abject failure. If one seemed to benefit one of the boys, it showed no benefit for the other. None showed enough benefit to use long-term, and we used only one supplement for more than three months. Before trying the supplements, I had called the Autism Research Institute, where the founder, Bernard Rimland, answered the phone, himself, on the second ring. He graciously discussed my hopes, dreams, and concerns about the supplements and advised me not to tell what we were trying to anyone who did not need to know. He said if someone expected the latest trial to answer all the problems, they would see only great things when they learned what we were doing. If someone believed it to be a waste of time, they would see only negative things from the moment we started.

Many of you will recognize this strategy as a sound research method. It drove a lot of people crazy, but I followed Dr. Rimland's advice the best I could. And it was great advice. Keeping this information to ourselves was a wonderful strategy with everyone except one teacher, Richard's fourth-grade teacher at the time. I couldn't put anything past her. She was a fantastic teacher and is still a valued friend. When Richard was in her class, I was substituting regularly within the same building. Every single time I tried something, she would show up at my classroom door with her hands on her hips and demand to know what we had done. It is a fantastic experience to have a teacher this in tune with your child. I hope all of you have a teacher or someone who supports you as she did in your life at some point.

Not everything we did in those days was from a textbook or clinical study. Much of what we tried stemmed from a desperate need to have a degree of normalcy while staying within our budget and attempting to incorporate the hopes and dreams we shared as a young couple trying to raise our children. We did a lot of social activities, which for us included mainly Boy Scouts and church. To encourage others to accept our boys' participation, we both volunteered for any activity the boys would participate in. The social activities of church and Scouts were usually beneficial to our sons, even though their participation was not always well received, as others thought we should have ensured they did not display behaviors associated with autism while they were there. While participating was challenging at times, we continued to join in the activities and many of the leaders, who were accepting and supportive of our work with the boys during this time, are still friends to this day.

People-First

During this learning process, I adopted the use of person-first language. Person-first language puts the person before the condition/disability, making someone an "individual who has autism" or a "woman who has diabetes" instead of an "autistic individual" or a "diabetic woman." Referring to individuals before the diagnosis focuses on the person, not the challenge. We do not discount their abilities before they have had the opportunity to try. I am not personally offended by someone who does not use this language, though I prefer it. Some people even find person-first language annoying. However, when the boys were in school, I realized educators and other professionals who made the effort to incorporate person-first language were more likely to put extra effort into their interventions. Like the teacher who noted every time we made a change that worked with Richard, and even some that didn't work, it was almost as if they were holding up a sign that said, "Here you will find a compassionate friend who does their best to provide a positive learning environment for your child." It was always a welcome sign, even if only in my head.

As a young mom, I had a hard time wrapping my brain around the ramifications of having two children who were on the spectrum. Person-first language gave me some relief. When working with someone who used this language, I felt I could focus on my children as the children I adored instead of on their autism. I latched onto the concept and enjoyed the reprieve provided me by thinking of myself simply as "Mom." Being an "autism mom" was a heavy burden, and I needed a break from that persona. I was hungry for anything that would make me feel like I was doing something right. Even though using person-first language worked wonders for me, I was surprised at the difference it made in other people when they used it. Even well-educated therapists and teachers have a completely different attitude towards the boys and our family when they, too, use person-first language. It made a noticeable difference in how in-tune the professionals were with our boys' needs. I quickly learned to gravitate towards working with professionals who made the extra effort.

Thankfully, the boys attended the same elementary and high school that my husband and I did, so quite a few people had known all of us for most of our lives through our school connections. When someone said something less than supportive in the presence of these loyal, beautiful people, my phone rang. We seemed to have our very own underground support network, for which I will be eternally grateful. I want to note that not once did our phone ring for someone to tell us an educator who used person-first language was being unsupportive or making hurtful comments. Even though, as I mentioned previously, I choose not to take offense when someone does not use person-first language, I prefer it because I have seen how this simple step changes attitudes toward providing a more inclusive atmosphere. I encourage you to give it a try. Make it a habit if it helps you and those listening to you.

Life with autism has brought our lives many highs and lows, but mainly a lot of love and deep relationships with our sons. We learned many things because we needed to stay on top of as much autism information as possible. For example, Richard was diagnosed as PDD-NOS, but nobody knew what that was, so we just said autism. In elementary the diagnostician came to us excited that there was a new autism diagnosis that would define Richard's diagnosis better, so she wanted to test him. We sat down to sign all the paperwork, and as she explained how wonderful it would be to change his diagnosis to Aspergers, I asked, "So how will this change his program at the school?" When they responded that it would not change anything, I put down the pen and told them no thank you. Until your child is the subject of one of these evaluations, you cannot possibly understand how much of an effect the process has on everyone. The DSM-V, The Diagnostic and Statistical Manual of Mental Disorders, Fifth Edition, (American Psychiatric Association 2013) solved our dilemma of reporting his diagnosis when they combined autism, PDD-NOS, and Aspergers into one diagnosis of Autism Spectrum Disorder. I learned early on to let go of the mom-/parent-guilt, do my best, and not look back. This adventure is not a sprint; it is a marathon. There are no quick answers to our challenges, only lots of little trials that eventually work out into routines we can maintain. The strategies that worked for us were taken on in increments, adding small portions of any new routines and then building upon those. Even now that our sons are adults, we make it a rule not to take on a challenge that will be so overwhelming it will fail just because of the complexity, and when we have failures, we chalk it up to experience and do not look back!

Chapter Two

Hopes and Dreams

Someday I want to see my boys living independently with no aid from others, completely autonomous. I see them managing their finances, insurance, nutrition, living environment, health, and social activity. My dream is for them to live self-sufficient, balanced lives. Wishing this for my sons makes me a typical mother, nothing more and nothing less. This book is about our family's journey to ensure our sons achieve this goal. I supply a record for those who care about my sons by writing this book. In the process, I want to pass along to you, the reader, some of the strategies we have learned and the mistakes we have made. While I learned these strategies to help facilitate my sons' journeys to independence, I also learned that these strategies are helpful for everyone, whether they have autism or not. If you are a professional reading this book, you may discover some insight into families affected by autism or any other special need and how they face challenges. If you are a parent, I hope you find some of our experiences helpful in working through your search for routines and habits that will pave the way for your child to develop the skills they need to be independent.

I view my most critical role as an autism advocate for my sons and others with autism. An autism advocate helps individualize strategies to meet the needs and goals of the people they work with. Obviously, advocating for individualized, person-centered strategies should be any parent's or professional's goal, whether the child/individual we are working with has autism, is typically developing, or has any other challenge. However, it is important to note that autism is not just a behavioral challenge for this country, but also a health challenge. In 2017, Autism Speaks published Autism and Health: A Special Report by Autism Speaks, Advances in Understanding and Treating the Health Conditions that Frequently Accompany Autism (Hirvikoski 2016; Guan 2017). This publication reports a life expectancy of thirty-six years for individuals with autism. How can that possibly be true? Unfortunately, this is what the data shows, though the CDC currently states thirty-nine as the age. Gastrointestinal disorders, hypertension, diabetes, obesity, sleep disorders, anxiety, and depression are higher in individuals with autism. Still, the most shocking is the likelihood of suicide at 433 percent compared to suicides in the general population (Croen 2014). The only acceptable response to these statistics is to find solutions that promote physical health, independence, mental health, and social connectedness. The need to address the health concerns listed applies to individuals with autism and those around them. Those with autism generally need some level of support past their eighteenth birthday; therefore, it only makes sense to take care of those with the diagnosis *and* those who support them. The need for support of both the individual and their caregivers becomes especially important due to the high rate of caregiver burnout experienced by parents and others providing long-term care.

Allow me to elaborate. Over the years, we have tried several strategies and treatments; however, we didn't get too extravagant, simply because we did not have the income to support expensive therapies. We also avoided any treatments we felt would interfere with the boys having as much of a typical childhood as possible. Our decisions about these treatments meant that over the years, we upset some of our social circle by not trying what they believed would be the answer for us. The person I was most likely to lean on for emotional support changed regularly. I talked to the psychologist about this phenomenon during the reassessment process for one of the boys. While I found it upsetting that I lost friends when I didn't take their advice, the psychologist saw it as nothing unusual. He encouraged me to get a counselor for myself. He explained that the amount of stress I went through daily was more than my friends experienced during a crisis. It comes down to the give and take of a relationship, and friendship just doesn't work unless both friends get something positive out of the relationship. Without realizing what I was doing, I leaned too hard on my friends, while not giving nearly as much back into the friendship as my friends gave me. It had nothing to do with whether I was a giving person. None of my friends had the exact intense need for a sounding board that I had. Why did I not just talk to other moms who had children with autism, you may ask? I didn't know any. As I mentioned earlier, the diagnosis at that point was extremely rare and this was long before the internet became so accessible. There were no electronic mailing lists, texting, or social media. No easy way to find support groups with people struggling along the same path we were. It was much more of a challenge back then to connect with people outside of your immediate circle.

Everyone needs emotional support, and those affected by autism are no exception. It's so easy to unconsciously put too much burden on your closest circle if you don't have a strong, like-minded support system. When dealing with your connections who don't share your struggles, whether they are friends, family, or acquaintances, it's important for everyone to respect boundaries. Looking back at the difficult moments in our lives, the need for boundaries in our support network seems much clearer, but because we didn't have connections then with people who shared our struggles, we were desperate and put too much on the personal community we did have. Not only did we need to respect boundaries, we also needed the support and respect from others that gave us room to make mistakes and create our own successes.

At times, I needed others who would listen without comment. Sometimes, I just needed encouragement. Other times, I needed advice. Balancing listening, support, and advice while not overtaxing relationships is difficult. For anyone reading this book, I wish for you, relationships that are honest enough to have frank conversations about boundaries and each other's current abilities to supply support. Every parent needs someone they can go to in times of crisis, even if that crisis is that your child has just upset you so much, you need someone to watch them for fifteen minutes while you calm down and regain your composure enough to be a good parent again. I only once took one of my children to someone else while I grabbed that fifteen-minute break to regain my composure. My child did not want a haircut and showed his displeasure by publicly slapping me. I was very thankful that day for a friend who could sit with my son while I calmed down and thought about going forward from that moment. While my policy is to do the best I can with the information I have at the time and not look back, I do look back on this one aspect of our lives and say I should have taken the counselor's advice and found a counselor for myself. It would have reduced the stress on friendships and our social networks and possibly even helped us find ways to incorporate family and friends more successfully into our journey.

One of the most important things we have learned in our autism adventure that brings us peace is to have a growth mindset. This attitude frees us from the burden of achieving perfection or facing utter failure. It frees us from the judgment of those who are disappointed that we don't take their advice. Rather than focusing on what is not going well, in a growth mindset every incremental improvement is a step worth celebrating and acknowledging. The idea is to work towards those gains, no matter how small, and believe improvement is possible. In a fixed mindset approach, we might believe the fate of a person's health and well-being is a set point that we cannot improve. Instead, in the growth-mindset, we applaud the effort as a success. Trying new foods requires significant effort and determination when the barrier is fear. These fears include the new food, itself, how it feels in the individual's mouth, how it tastes and smells, and the reactions of those at the table if the person does not eat or like it. When the effort is always encouraged and celebrated, eating with those who support the process becomes a safe place where curiosity and new experiences are the expected reaction from everyone. Using this method also establishes boundaries that allow both the parents and the child with autism to work towards their individual goals. While the parent may want calm meals where they can relax while everyone eats nutritious food, the person with autism may simply want food they feel comfortable eating.

The Challenge

With that in mind, let's delve a little further into one of the most important foundations of a growth mindset, truth. When Richard was in second grade, during an IEP (Individualized Education Plan) meeting, the diagnostician reported to us that while testing Richard had expressed that he had no friends. I asked when Richard had made this statement, thinking maybe he had a bad week. The diagnostician told me he had given this answer to a test eighteen months prior. Eighteen months. In the IEP which followed that test, the fact that my son was lonely was not mentioned. I would have remembered. After asking why the diagnostician did not report it the previous year, she told me, "We don't tell everything to the parents all at once. It's a lot to handle." I must have gone from pale to red because she immediately said, "We can't do that with you, can we?" My response was, "No, I need it hard and cold. If you only give me half the problem, I can only work on half the solution." From that moment, it has been my motto to seek the whole truth of the challenges we face to improve the boys' lives.

A growth mindset addresses *truths*. Praise all efforts, but tell the truth. If your individual is not eating a balanced enough diet to prevent future health issues, that is a truth that needs to be addressed. If your individual makes comments at mealtime that upset others at the table, this interaction needs to be redirected to another habit. Those challenges require effort and improvement, which should receive praise at every step, while not capping their abilities with statements like "you will never" or "you will always." Every person can improve, whether we are talking about fitness, nutritional balance, or social skills, to name a few areas. Using a growth mindset, predictability, and positive habits, we work through plans to improve health, social skills, and life skills on the road to independence. The challenges and emotions we see as these individuals work on expanding their accepted foods are only the tip of the iceberg. There are many other difficulties, which we can only guess at and imagine.

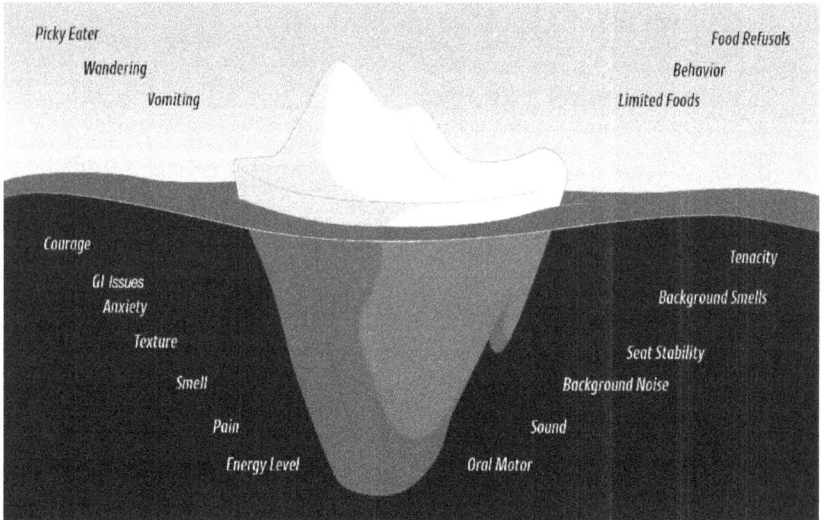

Figure 2-1
James Lemons III©

In Seven Habits for Highly Effective People, Steven Covey (Covey 2004) encourages us to begin with the end in mind, advice which I mirror in this book. I would like to see the end result being individuals eating well-balanced meals that support their health while honoring their preferences for flavors, satisfying their hunger, and having joyful, stress-free meals filled with pleasant memories. I would like to see as many individuals with autism as possible living independently, planning well-balanced meals, and preparing meals without help. I feel it is also essential for them to have the ability to work through the challenges that occur because they have learned how to approach and conquer these difficulties in their home in a way that fosters self-advocacy and the skills needed to tend to the daily tasks necessary for living autonomously. Mealtimes, whether everyone gathers at a table or somewhere else, are the perfect place to address these challenges as a team and begin to see what is under the iceberg tip.

The advantages of eating meals together have been researched and recounted for a long time. I recognize that eating meals with someone with autism is a challenge, but I also see it as an opportunity for the many benefits families facing autism need.

One day while we were eating, Jason said, "The smoke alarms were going off today." We continued with our meal, then he said the smoke alarms had gone off while he was in Ms. Ornelas' room. Since he mentioned it twice, he had my attention. Jason shared details about his day only when he was stressed and something was wrong. Mentioning the details of his day was a cry for help, so we asked him some follow up questions and figured out that though the alarms were going off, the students and staff had not evacuated. The next day, I contacted Ms. Ornelas and found out the alarms had been malfunctioning and, indeed, were sounding throughout the day. After each alarm, the office announced, "Disregard the smoke alarms." Disregard? Jason could not fathom disregarding the smoke alarms, so, he was not doing well in this situation. We requested an IEP meeting to address how the school would handle future fire alarms with Jason. If our family had not been having meals together, we would not have been able to avert the situation quickly.

Different Perspectives

We also discovered during family dinner how a well-intentioned, but misguided, interdisciplinary team was trying to fit Richard, our oldest, into a mold that didn't fit his likes and interests. The team had decided he needed to be more "macho," so I agreed to let them teach him some more "masculine" skills. However, we did not define or give input into what skills were necessary for this to happen. It turns out they felt he wasn't manly enough because he didn't talk about sports, so they taught him to discuss the latest Cowboys football game and then wanted him to practice at home. Dutifully, he came home and tried to start a conversation about football, which went exactly nowhere. Why? James and I aren't sports fans. Furthermore, we aren't fans of watching TV much at all. When we asked why the sudden desire to talk about football, we found out his interdisciplinary team's idea of macho was having sports conversations. A topic which held no importance in our home. Our macho concept was more about camping skills, courteousness to others, and the ability to help with house maintenance, so I encourage you to learn from our mistakes. When deciding the goals that bring someone closer to independence, consider their personal and social preferences. We all see life through our own lens. It is vital to consider what that lens looks like for individuals within their social network. All interventions should center around what best serves the individual's interests, needs, and wishes. Let me say that again. *All interventions should center around what best serves the individual's interests, needs, and wishes.* It's easy when you feel you are drowning to look only at the immediate situation and forget that your individual with autism is just that. An individual. *A person*. And each person has their own likes, needs, goals, and desires. While a person who has autism may need more direction and help in everyday matters, they do not lose their personality. With that in mind, setting goals and intervention strategy is an area where I find stories to be very helpful. When making goals, write down how you see the attainment of these goals playing out in the future, and if someone is proposing a goal, ask them to tell you a story about how they see the future if this goal is reached.

Having a Hard Time

Here's an important truism: Individuals with autism do not give you a hard time; they have a hard time. In general, I think diagnosticians, psychologists, educators, and treatment teams who worked with my boys truly had their best interest in mind. However, those professionals didn't know my children, our home life, our family needs and likes, nor our day-to-day routines, and there certainly wasn't the sheer amount of information and training available to professionals who work with autism as there is today. A speech therapist once told me a child's swallowing issues were behavioral. She insisted that she was swallowing incorrectly on purpose to get attention from the parents. I asked her, "Could you do that? Could you swallow every single swallow of your life incorrectly just to get attention?" I do not believe it is realistic to think a child with autism is repeating a behavior consistently just to annoy us. We tend to say, "Stop that," without suggesting a more acceptable behavior. I always give an alternative when trying to stop a behavior. The child needs to know what to do instead of the unwanted behavior. If you do not do this, they may pick another habit you find just as annoying or even more so. I believe it is better to teach our individuals how to work through difficult situations, enabling them to handle similar situations on their own later without the family, therapist, or educators there to help.

Our family has focused much of our efforts on promoting the ability to work through challenges autonomously. For our sons to become genuinely independent, this is an essential skill. I don't want to see them eating each and every bite of food someone puts on their plates any more than I want them bending to peer pressure in every situation. I want them to be able to figure out their hunger and fullness cues, along with their likes and dislikes while at the same time accepting and consuming enough of a nutritionally diverse diet to support good health. It is also essential for them to be respectful and courteous if they are unwilling to eat the food someone offers them. Furthermore, it is essential for them to learn to set boundaries with others.

Our interactions at the table are a testing ground for what will work in other relationships. I consider the nutrition implications of setting boundaries around food fundamental, but the essential skill here is not the nutrition piece. Boundary-setting is crucial to establishing limits with others, and knowing how to read and respect boundaries that others need is vital to developing strong relationships. It is not only the ability to make decisions about oneself and define limits with others by focusing on habits that promote health and good relationships, but also a bidirectional lesson we learn by seeing and interpreting the physical reactions and facial expressions of those we interact with. It goes much deeper than picking food preferences and includes limits on how we expect others to speak to us and how close we allow them physically, and the same can be said for respecting the boundaries of others. Everyone benefits from learning to read the reactions of other people. These are hard lessons, and like in everything else, those with autism need more practice than others. They also probably need exaggerated reactions from those close to them to understand this lesson. Around the table, everyone is close enough to see the physical responses of their tablemates. If someone says something that makes another cry, they are right there, face-to-face to see it. The same is true if they say or do something that makes someone happy. Because individuals with autism are often not strong at making inferences, it is helpful when we say aloud how we feel to aid in verifying that our individual's interpretation is correct.

Like every young family, we started our journey with hopes and dreams of bright futures for our children that included happy, healthy lives. We still have those dreams. Our boys' futures may look slightly different than we first imagined, but they are successful and happy. We have worked hard to ensure our sons have had opportunities to live their lives in a way that gives them joy while preparing them for that someday when they will live separately from us. With encouragement, they have developed relationships outside of the family and have felt free to explore their own interests. To that point, Jason has developed an interest in many sports despite our own lack of interest in them. How your family navigates this journey is as individual as you and your child are. May your expedition through life be filled with joy as you and they follow their aspirations and visions for the future.

Chapter Three

Trust and Joy

    My favorite memories of meals together include holidays at my grandparents where there wasn't enough room for the children at the table, so all of us kids knelt on the floor in front of a chair, the seat becoming our table. Easter gatherings with cousins, where nobody monitored what I did or did not eat, were particularly special to me. We simply had fun and enjoyed each other's company. Later, as an adult, I enjoyed hosting gatherings in my own home for my extended family. Communal meals are an important part of relationship building, and those moments gathered around a table should be joyful, not stressful. Even while modifying my diet and the foods I prepare to accommodate my own health needs and the individual food plans of my family, I still savor mealtimes. I believe everyone should be able to relish their food and their relationships with those who share the table. For those with limited choices due to medical issues, sensory reasons, or social anxiety, it is still vital to join in with others, even when we do not want to eat the food they are eating or maybe have not even tried the foods they are eating. Enjoyment is essential for developing healthy relationships with both food and those around us. Joy and fellowship are my primary goals when I host a dinner. As we nourish our bodies with food, we also nourish ourselves with happy relationships and a special time for strengthening bonds with friends and family.

What does joy at mealtime look like to you? Dictionary.com defines joy as "a source or cause of keen pleasure or delight." Do you achieve this by planning and preparing meals together, then eating delicious food as the family shares their day's highs and lows? Some people may enjoy eating their favorite foods quietly in the company of the ones they love or maybe, even, all alone.

My view of joy at mealtime has evolved over the years. I love creating an environment where everyone at the table has fun being present and participating in friendly conversation. Individuals *choose* to eat the food rather than *comply* with someone else's wishes. Everyone enjoys eating the food prepared and has no fear of being pressured to eat something that makes them feel uncomfortable. Trying or declining unfamiliar foods and recipes according to their comfort level is not stress-inducing. Everyone is encouraged to discuss what they do or do not like about their food, and their willingness to eat those foods is respected and encouraged. The joy in these experiences comes from a combination of eating food we find pleasurable and the fellowship with our tablemates. Creating joy is where we should start when developing goals for eating and wellness.

The Essential Ingredient

Trust is an essential ingredient for achieving joy during meals. As Stephen Covey discusses in his book, The Speed of Trust (Covey 2018), building trust is like having a bank account for the relationship. Applying Covey's analogy to the food offered during meals, you deposit trust in the account each time you show there will be no consequences for disliking a food and no pressure to eat it. Conversely, a withdrawal from the account is made if you try to sneak in food or pressure the individual to eat. The person who hid the food has not been honest; they have not shown confidence that the individual will attempt to try the food, and they have not honored the fear that is felt by the individual regarding this food. Honoring the fear felt when trying new foods allows that individual to relax, trust their tablemates, and feel joy during meals. An individual who trusts that the food they are eating will not cause any physical reaction or aversion and knows it will be acceptable for them to refuse that food has no fear. Once, when I was talking to an adult with autism about trying new foods, she told me, "If you ever try to sneak something into my food without telling me, I will never trust you again."

Trust needs to be kept in order to increase the variety of foods and the diversity of nutrition and balance in someone's eating plan. Every person does not need to like each food offered to eat a balanced diet, nor does it happen overnight. It is a process over time of finding foods that bring nutritional balance while also acknowledging food preferences. Families will need to use creativity to find foods that fit the unique sensory profile of their individual and the nutritional balance needed.

Food exploration is important for expanding the variety and number of food choices your child confidently eats. Using sameness and predictability in knowing what is expected and allowed helps ease these fears. Consistency develops confidence. If there is to be a new food, ingredient, or a change in the place settings at the meal, discuss it openly. Challenge one fear at a time, whether the fear is of new foods or a change in the environment. If the setting of the meal is changed by introducing a different placemat, plate color, or which family members are present at the meal, there should be no surprises in the food that is served, even if it means for those occasions, separate food is provided for your child. The same is true for the reverse situation. If introducing a new food, the surroundings should be consistent. Limit challenges to one at a time while keeping the same rules in place daily, allowing the individual the power to reject or the curiosity to eat new foods only if they are comfortable enough. They can relax and enjoy their food and the relationships formed at the table while developing new skills such as conversation and appropriate social interaction, elements as crucial to emotional and mental health as nutritious foods are to the body. The tone must remain optimistic, but there also must be transparency to keep the conversations positive. Trust only exists when there is transparency. Trust-building extends to all members of the family and those present at meals will have various requirements to be part of this critical relationship. For the adults and siblings at the table, this may include knowing the person with autism will decline to eat an offered food using a method that has already been agreed upon as acceptable.

Methods to decline food might include placing the rejected food on a saucer, verbally saying no thank you, or spitting disliked food into a napkin and carrying it to the trash. These preplanned, socially acceptable ways of saying no will keep the mealtime pleasant for all. The good news is through honoring your individual's choices while creatively adding foods and skills one step at a time, it is possible that eventually your individual can eat alongside others, enjoying nutritious meals that meet their health needs in a situation that meets their relational needs. All of this is definitely worth the effort, as my own family has proven out.

It is an understatement to say developing joy and trust during mealtimes with autism is not always easy, but it is an excellent place to begin changing the outlook on mental and physical health. One of the most frustrating experiences for me as a parent was when another person would define what I should expect regarding the potential of my children. It wasn't unusual for me to be told that my family would be much better off if I accepted that there would be certain things the boys would never be able to do and to quit putting the family under stress by trying to achieve something which that person believed was unachievable. That's the epitome of a fixed mindset. I never put limits on my sons' potential, and I believed in encouraging them to get as close to their personal goals as possible, so we moved forward and continue to do so.

I feel the same about realistic goals for one's health. Nobody should put limits on another person. Just as a runner can improve their skills and endurance with practice until they reach the goal of becoming a marathon runner, a person with autism can train themselves, by working on a limited set of specific goals, to gradually increase their comfort in eating with others and eating a balanced diet. While a fixed mindset would say this isn't possible, a growth mindset would believe that improving long-term health by making incremental changes is possible, viewing each small victory as worthy of celebration all along the way. Priorities, however, should be reevaluated from time to time to reaffirm they are appropriate, and the family is not being overwhelmed with rigid routines governing every action throughout the day. The relationship with food and those present at mealtime takes precedence over other objectives when developing targets for eating. For someone with sensory issues, hunger and fullness cues may be confused with the need to use food to self-soothe due to stress, boredom, or reflux pain. Those with a fatalistic attitude would believe such a situation could not be changed because sensory issues are so hard to overcome. This is an inaccurate viewpoint, however, as there are mitigations that can be introduced. When needing comfort, a menu of other options that includes alternatives to food may need to be developed. Positive relationships with food are essential for many reasons, including the overlap between autism and eating disorders.

The Apple Test

My friend and eating disorder guru, Jessica Setnick of www.understandingnutrition.com, uses this test to determine hunger versus boredom, stress, or other motivators to eat when not really hungry. Whether someone is going for second helpings, eating a large portion of food at a meal, or is eating a snack, they should ask themselves, "If that were an apple, would I eat it?" If the answer is no, then they probably need something else besides food. The "something else" has endless possibilities. Do they need to:

- Take a nap
- Call a friend
- Color
- Do something productive
- Seek some sensory input like punching a pillow or wrapping themselves in a weighted blanket
- Write in their journal
- Work with tools
- Make something creative
- Draw

Other needs that beg for attention instead of food are endless. For individuals on the spectrum, I would investigate potential sensory activities. Chewing, especially if it is something crunchy, can fill a need for those seeking sensory input, but many other possibilities also fill this need including chopping food, pounding on something, or any other activity that might include strenuous use of muscles. For those that may not be fans of apples, I substitute a different produce into the question, for example if that were a piece of celery, carrot, or orange would I eat it?

While I hope the strategies I write about will help anyone trying to improve their health and lead an autonomous life, the reality is that feeding a child with sensory and picky eating issues is particularly challenging, leaving families stressed. The truth is it is not just nutrition that affects current and future health status, but also the stress level within the home. In 1998, the Journal of Preventive Medicine published the Adverse Childhood Experiences Study, which showed a correlation between specific experiences and a higher incidence of disease, depression, risky behaviors, early death, and attempted suicide (Felitti, 1998). These experiences included verbal abuse, physical abuse, substance abuse in the home, family dysfunction, mental illness, and mothers who have suffered abuse. This study emphasizes the long-term effects of growing up in a home where adverse events within the home have long-term effects on physical and mental health. These elements are already known to be more prevalent in the lives of those who have autism. It is not a far leap to conclude that reducing stress is essential to improving the lives of those with autism and their family members. Parents of children who have autism feel intense pressure from many directions. Finding ways to make mealtimes joyful and less stressful is a good place to start reducing adverse experiences in the home.

It is hard to feel joy during meals, however, when you are worried about everything you are supposed to do for your child. To ensure a child is growing at a proper rate, sufficient food has to be eaten. Parents feel pressured to serve all the food groups and ensure their child eats them to provide the essential vitamins and minerals. While balancing these feats, parents are also trying to teach their child table manners, social skills, and table conversation appropriate for school and grandma's house.

The Adverse Childhood Events study speaks to me on a very personal level. If I put on my parent's hat, I can see I need to protect our home environment from being toxic. My husband and I have always worked hard to be on the same page and present a united front for our children, but now that those children are adults, unity in purpose and respectful treatment of each other is a family discussion. If I put on my professional hat, I want to ensure any recommendations I provide to families I consult with will work within that family's particular living environment. A child's caregiver may not be a parent or even a relative. There may be several individuals in the home with challenging situations. Having a child with autism does not make you and your family immune to the range of challenges the world presents. There may be others in the home with health issues and there will be times that life just happens. Relationships change, as do jobs and financial obligations. Nobody gets to live in a bubble while they work on feeding challenges. The most critical intervention I work on may be helping a family move towards pleasant mealtimes. Providing a vehicle for a family to have a peaceful moment where everyone can relax is sometimes more important than nutritional balance or perfect meals. I encourage parents to protect the time they spend together during meals as an oasis of family harmony. While expanding the variety of food eaten may improve health, tranquility at meals also has a positive effect on health.

For all children, it is imperative to preserve relationships and positive experiences, and communal mealtime needs to be a top priority when setting goals. The advantages that come from eating together include healthier food choices, better long-term health, stronger relationships, increased school performance, and improved mental health. Individuals who have autism receive these same benefits from family mealtimes; however, they need more practice to achieve mastery than their typically developing peers. Strained or challenging mealtimes affect everyone, but autism magnifies stress in all areas of life and can especially be a barrier to joy during meals. The devotion to sameness seen in autism may result in many problems. Tantrums can stem from the wrong plate or utensil, or from food being cut up when the individual wanted whole pieces. Frustration and tears may spring from food that is round rather than square or has an unexpected texture. Understandably, meals are more comfortable and pleasant when predictability is maintained by serving the same foods on the same plates while using the same placemats. However, believing everyone will always maintain this degree of sameness is unrealistic. At times there may be no joy at all in the meals. Adults and children know their tablemates' reactions may be unpleasant when the precise mealtime routine changes and dread it. It is not difficult to see why many families are willing to provide precisely the food and environment to ensure a calmer, quieter, more pleasant meal.

Behavior Is Communication

In working toward more pleasant mealtimes, or any other goal, it is vital to remember that the behavior of your individual is communication and all interventions should be based on your child's behavior. One of the most profound lessons I learned when my children were young was to watch what they *were* doing, not what they were *not* doing. When evaluating chewing and swallowing issues, it helps to look at the gross motor skills of sitting up, crawling, and walking. The ability to chew follows those skills. Children who have not developed gross motor skills sufficiently to crawl or walk will not be ready to progress to chewing foods with more complex textures.

Interestingly enough, this works in reverse. Someone who has lost the ability to sit, crawl, or walk due to aging or an accident may lose the ability to chew and swallow. Behaviors communicate issues or problems. Acknowledging that the individual's fears or behavioral struggles are a form of communication builds trust in their relationship with the parents. Consequently, it adds joy when parents and children can read each other's verbal and non-verbal cues.

I've also learned to watch for clues such as a person's eyes looking at the food and then looking for a place to dispose of it. Are they moving food into their mashed potatoes before taking a bite? Or are they watching everyone at the table to see who is not eating food because they want to sneak a bite when carrying the plate to the sink? Watching what others are leaving on their plate may indicate not getting full enough from what they have eaten off their own plate. They may also be watching someone at the table to see if they, themselves, are being watched. They might be concerned about that person's judgment of what they are or are not eating. The individual might be more willing to try a food or eat more of a food if someone they admire likes it. All of these behaviors can be indicators of their likes, dislikes, and needs.

My husband grew up eating meatloaf made with oatmeal. I gag at the texture of oatmeal. He tried every recipe combination he could find. He even took the oatmeal and ran it through the blender to make it a powder, then used it as an ingredient. I thought I was doing an excellent job hiding my texture issue, but he eventually turned to me and said, "You are gagging on that. Drinking water after every bite and hiding your coughing doesn't change the fact you're gagging." He was correct and changed to a recipe with breadcrumbs. Did I mention it is not only our boys who struggle with food texture issues? Nope, sometimes the parents do, as well.

The other issue that needs to be addressed here is that of

pediatric feeding disorders. Remembering the above truism, that behavior is communication, a child's difficulty with feeding is a communication of a problem that needs to be addressed. One of the first recognized traits of autism is the refusal to eat or difficulty eating. While each person is different, it is not unusual for a child who will later be diagnosed with autism to have difficulties feeding on the breast or bottle in infancy. As the child ages, challenges with the suck-swallow-breath coordination needed for liquid consumption may indicate oral-motor issues that can benefit from working with a feeding therapist. Before increasing the variety of food eaten, oral-motor therapists should evaluate the individual's mechanical problems with chewing and swallowing, if there seems to be a problem.

When my middle son was in his thirties, a dentist told me he needed to do a gum graft because Jason was lip-tied, and we needed to change our plan for some of his dental work since he had a high palette. When I said, "Well, of course he is," the dentist first looked at me like I was crazy, then asked me to explain. I had been fortunate enough to work with both an occupational therapist and a speech and language pathologist who were aware of this phenomenon in individuals with autism. Just as an oral-motor therapist had educated me, I had the opportunity to educate the dentist.

While researching for this book, I found further confirmation that individuals with autism have a higher incidence of physical anomalies like high palates. My son did have challenges associated with high palates and oral tissue ties like lip ties. These physical issues caused him difficulty with prolonged nursing sessions as an infant and, as he matured, he had speech issues, eating challenges, growth challenges, and difficulty cleaning his teeth properly. However, we did not recognize those issues as communication of a need at the time.

Additionally, many individuals with autism or other developmental disorders experience pain or discomfort from reflux and sensory issues. Difficulty swallowing or chewing could be the basis for fear. The ability to eat food and drink liquids is a skill that I never considered until I started working with children in an early intervention program. Like most people, it never occurred to me that this could be difficult to learn. But, for many children learning skills related to eating requires some help. Children who resist being fed or moving on to the next expected texture may have a structural or sensory issue. I have seen many children who were referred to me for a behavioral issue with food, and when we dug deeper and watched what the child was doing, we found the problem was medical or developmental. Suppose an individual is chewing more like a chipmunk in the front of their mouth. Chewing should look more like a cow with a visible jaw rotation. An oral-motor therapist should evaluate the ability to chew and swallow correctly. Understanding that your individual may not have the words or the ability to express a physical need and seeing their behavior as a form of communication can help you and the professionals on their therapy team mitigate, or even overcome, some of the challenges that present themselves as your individual matures.

Dealing with Other People's Expectations

Families enjoy having a relaxed meal with free-flowing conversation, but achieving this nirvana when you finally sit down to eat may involve the stress of going to three places, including two different fast-food restaurants, just to ensure the individual with autism has two foods they will eat during the meal. I have done this, as have many other parents. Additionally, if feeding disorders, allergies, or other health issues are present, your individual may have even more specific needs that create stress. Judgment by friends, family, and healthcare professionals about the food a child with autism eats is more the norm than the exception, and parents often feel trapped between the stress of a social network that disapproves and the ever-demanding health needs of their child. Desperate parents do whatever they can to get through the day. The name of the game is always survival. Surmounting challenges happens one day, an hour, or a minute at a time. Parents need support from friends, relatives, and professionals to overcome these challenges. Unfortunately, those within the families' social network are also frequently overwhelmed by autism, leaving the families feeling unsupported and isolated.

When our boys were small, holidays were incredibly stressful. They would eat very little food or even none. We learned to bring the boys' favorite foods to contribute to the meal. When they ate, it was usually only the food we brought, but they refused to eat any food on some occasions. Their resistance to eating other foods was always a topic of conversation. Grandparents were especially concerned. The boys took many years of gradual progress to find comfort during holiday meals.

I think most of us parents feel we must be the only people in the world who feel this way or there must be something wrong with our parenting skills if we are having "this" experience. So, I want to acknowledge some of the experiences that I feel are pretty common for parents of children with autism. To be fair, I'll include both good and bad experiences. The following is a short list compared to the reality we face, but it will give you a small taste of the difficulties and the wins.

- Your social network "forgets" to notify you of events.
- There are additional requirements for your family to participate in an event.
- Someone close to you will suddenly be unable to cope with the challenges you share with them.
- You will become close to someone in your network because they are an active listener and offer helpful insight into your challenges.
- Someone you thought would support you and your children through any challenge *will* do exactly that.
- Someone you thought would support you and your children through any challenge will not.
- Someone in your social network will have what they believe is the absolute answer to all your challenges and will exert extreme pressure for you to follow their recommendations, no matter the cost.
- Someone in your social network will openly inform you they can no longer be supportive because you are not taking their advice.

- People you barely know will offer a surprisingly generous gift of support. Note: only accept offers that genuinely work for your family
- Family, friends, and social network will tell you they admired how well you handled parenting a child with autism, even though they never told you this when the challenge was the heaviest.
- An adult will expect a higher level of compliance and behavior than is realistic from your child who has autism.

Walking a Tight Rope

In a home affected by autism, parents feel pressure from family, friends, and professionals such as doctors and educators. One of the things that amazed me when our yearly Individual Education Plan (IEP) meeting rolled around was how detailed my children's evaluations were. When the diagnostician started talking about the angle in which my child held his hands, I wanted to scream. What parent would ever expect to have their child evaluated that closely? It's no wonder that achieving joy under this kind of strain becomes difficult. To ask a family to teach a child how to sit at a table and eat their food in a way society finds socially appropriate while supporting this child's sensory struggles and lack of understanding of social cues is an enormous thing to ask at the end of a rough day. Having said this, families can achieve predictable habits and view their child's behavior as the communication of a problem that can be solved and improved over time, creating trust and joy in their mealtime routines, but it is a challenge.

In addressing these challenges, some strategies employed by various therapy programs involve teaching children to comply with every request to eat the foods presented. I am uncomfortable with this didactic method. To permanently include more diverse foods in meals, the individual must *choose* to eat it rather than *comply* with the request or insistence that they eat every food. If they are only eating it because someone exerts pressure, they will stop when that pressure goes away. This could result in learning to eat every bite offered while not learning to respond to hunger and fullness cues. Additionally, every individual must learn to set boundaries in all areas of their lives by being able to decline when they don't want to do something. Saying no to food when you are full is one of the earliest boundaries we all learn to set.

Teaching children that it is okay to say no at times must be practiced at home to be able to successfully navigate social situations like bullying, unwanted touching, or predatory advances. When we can make a choice, we feel heard and that our needs and preferences have been honored. We feel valued as a person. Requiring total compliance does the opposite. Enjoying eating from all the food groups as an election rather than a requirement will ensure delicious, healthy food choices when selecting what to eat independently. Conversely, coercion will not transfer to independent meal planning and preparation. It is important to note here that learning boundaries is a two-way street. Having predetermined alternatives and preset rules for when alternatives are acceptable is important. When someone does not want one of the foods served at mealtimes, preparing a completely different meal should not be one of the alternatives. I make it a policy to include at least two foods that everyone will eat in my meal plans. If only one or no foods that an individual will eat are available, there will be resistance. Every person must have enough food to eat until they are full at every meal.

Pressure-Free Zone at Mealtime

Pressure with feeding and mealtimes is a reality for most individuals with autism. Studies on feeding issues and picky eating consistently show that eighty percent or more of families are concerned about their child's eating habits. The stress can be immense. At the beginning of our journey, our meals were not stress-free. I wish we had learned about growth mindsets early, but we did not. We made lots of mistakes along the way. Our pediatrician very adamantly insisted I offer the same food to my child every meal until he ate it. Like most people raised in the 1960s, we were taught children sit at the table until they finish their meal. With our upbringing, this professional advice didn't seem strange, so we set into motion the plan the pediatrician said would cure all our feeding woes. I prepared mashed potatoes because every kid likes mashed potatoes, don't they? The pediatrician said when our child got hungry, he would eat them. So, the first night, I offered him my best-prepared mashed potatoes. He quickly ate the chicken and gelatin accompanying the potatoes and asked if he could be excused. I explained that we were working on eating vegetables and that these potatoes would reappear until he ate them. He said "okay" and went off to play. The potatoes reappeared at breakfast and then at lunch, and each time he looked at me and asked, "Is this all there is?" When I responded yes to this he asked, "May I be excused?" After three meals of this routine, I gave up. Obviously, this was not the solution that was going to work for our family. I hope our journey from fixed-mindset eating to a growth-mindset approach entertains you. I also hope it gives you permission to laugh at us and maybe yourselves sometimes and, maybe, even inspires you to be creative in your strategies to help someone with autism reach their most independent, self-sufficient, well-nourished self. But I must warn you, while *you* may be able laugh at some of the difficulties and challenges, doctors, relatives, and friends do not tend to laugh and, often, seem to think parents are not trying hard enough.

That perception, that parents are not trying hard enough, is just not correct. The most excellent parents can have difficulty feeding their children for various reasons, including prematurity, reflux, food allergies, oral-motor issues, and autism, to name a few. These children are not born with an instruction manual that says your child has (this problem) and, therefore, you will need to do (a, b, c) to feed him properly and have an enjoyable experience while you are doing it. Learning what each child needs during feeding and all other growth experiences is a dance. Parents and children will have to learn to take turns leading that dance, how each should respond to the other, and what boundaries need to be respected.

As I have talked to parents of children who have autism, and in my own experience, I have found a minimal variety of food consumed in households with autism. It is not unusual for parents to tell me their child eats only chicken nuggets from McDonald's, fries from Wendy's, and starchy snacks like Goldfish crackers or Teddy Grahams. Often these are the parents I mentioned in the section titled *Dealing with Other People's Expectations*, who are more than willing to drive to several fast-food restaurants to get those few special foods their child will eat. This shows me these things:

- The parents will go out of their way, literally, to multiple locations to get their child to eat from more than one food group.
- New foods will be challenging for sensory reasons or outright fear of some foods.
- The child's gut microbiome may be ill-prepared to digest a large variety of food due to an earlier lack of exposure to those foods. Therefore, introducing new foods should be done in small amounts.
- Malnutrition and balancing the diet to have the diversity of nutrients needed to support good health is a priority due to the lack of or excess intake of nutritional elements.
- Assessment of medical issues like oral-motor, gastrointestinal, and swallowing issues must be ruled out or addressed.

People find comfort in the ability to predict what will happen. We like knowing the light will come on when we flip the switch, and that we can access the Internet by turning on our computers or just touching our smartphones. The same is true for eating. We all enjoy eating our favorite foods during holidays or at our favorite restaurants. When the menu is changed, we are disappointed. If the change is significant enough, we may go to another restaurant immediately or plan to eat somewhere else the next time we go out. Adults often make loud statements of disapproval, make the waitstaff miserable, or short-change the tip. Children cannot do these things, especially if the unwanted change is in their homes; however, they can use their behavior to communicate their frustration with the lack of predictability. It is the job of the caregivers and professionals to figure out what those behaviors are communicating. Individuals with sensory issues often like prepackaged crunchy foods, which is very predictable. Your child's favorite crackers and cookies are the same every time they come out of the box; however, fruits or vegetables are different. Their texture can be crunchy, mushy, soft, or grainy (to name a few), but it will not be the same every time. For a child with autism, the inconsistent qualities of foods may fill their hearts with fear that triggers unwanted behavior such as meltdowns, crying, food refusals, or spitting food out.

My big "Aha!" moment in making the connection between the ability to predict a devotion to the familiar and not wanting to try new foods, came when I watched a TED Talk titled "How Brains Learn to See," Pawan Sinha gave in 2009. I later realized it had been well established that those with autism have difficulty predicting. They are great historians but lousy predictors. That makes perfect sense as to why trying new foods is difficult. It is scary if you cannot predict how food will taste or feel in your mouth. Fear is preventing the individual from trying new foods, so they eat the foods they know and like. Our challenge as families and professionals is to make it safe for these individuals to try new foods.

This requires predictable responses from those offering the food, however, yelling at or punishing someone when they do not eat a food only creates more fear of trying novel foods. If the "rules" allow them to take one bite and say no or provide an acceptable way to remove the food from their mouth while the others at the table support their efforts, they will be more likely to put it in their mouth to start with. This consistent reaction supplies the sameness they crave while supplying a method to slowly alter the routine and scaffold in new food choices, social skills, and table skills in a fear-free zone. Some food play, which is discussed in the following paragraphs, may be allowed; however, I do not recommend every meal become a therapy session. Everyone deserves downtime from constantly being on-task, including both the child and the parents. Regularly, there should be meals where everyone eats food they find acceptable, and nobody has to prompt someone else to experience new food.

    I encourage trying all the food presented, but I have redefined the word 'try.' Trying a new food may initially mean that the individual ate their preferred food without throwing a tantrum because a food they will not eat was on the table. Trying can progress to putting it on their plate but not eating it, then interacting with the food by cutting, mashing, or smelling it before taking an extra-tiny bite that they can spit out in a predetermined routine. The next step might advance to carrying the food in their hand to the trash or helping to clean the table and dispose of or store the leftovers.

When food play is incorporated, it should include scenarios that are interesting to the child. Some examples are:

- pretending to be a dinosaur eating trees, which are, in reality, broccoli
- pretending green peas in the gravy of potatoes are turtles in a pond
- using vegetables as cars or trains
- using fruit instead of a chip or other favorite food, but only as a vehicle to eat the preferred food

These food play activities can make the meal much less scary for the individual. Trying unfamiliar foods does not necessarily include putting them in the mouth, swallowing them, and finishing the serving. Praise the effort, even if the only thing they did was sit next to someone who was eating a food they did not like without making too much fuss. It is also a good idea to have them handle the food during preparation or supply ways to be exposed to the smell. Activities like cutting or mashing food will help someone become familiar with the scent and texture. Other strategies for introducing the sensory aspects of food before asking someone to taste it can be found in the chapter on sensory exploration of food.

Creating predictable habits using a growth mindset as you offer novel foods is the key to making it safe to try them without fear. The variety of foods eaten can improve by adding one food at a time. Remember, progress does not need to be fast to make a difference. In educational and therapy circles, the term scaffolding is used to mean breaking large chunks of information into approachable, supported levels. With this in mind, scaffold the steps of introducing new foods into manageable tasks that move from demonstration to cooperation, with caregiver support gradually being withdrawn along the way, until the happy end-goal of independent task completion is reached. This allows for increasing familiarity with, and hopefully acceptance of, a wider variety of foods. Allowing the individual to slowly explore then assist with meal preparation is much more likely to result in enjoyment of the new food at mealtime, while preserving the individual's sense of personal choice.

The parent may need to help cut or mash the food initially and then encourage more independent manipulation as time passes, such as fork and knife skills or food preparation. By integrating learning into real-life experiences like food preparation, your individual can see a connection between the skill and its purpose. The experience also supplies a way of showing competence level. Demonstrating abilities can show which skills need improvement before the individual can plan, prepare, and cook sufficiently to manage their nutritional needs without someone hovering, ready to help.

We all learn more effectively in chunks rather than in mass quantities of information. Allow your individual with autism to learn one skill at a time, then use each repeatedly so that it is cemented into long-term memory. While I start the process by using abilities needed to support a balanced diet, these strategies work for learning all skills, from teeth brushing to meal planning to household chores. All are necessary to obtain the brass ring of living a self-sufficient life.

Chapter Four

Meal Planning

Meal planning for busy families with picky eaters can be a challenge. Our family is no exception. When it comes to food, we can agree on chocolate cake. Specifically, a Betty Crocker yellow cake mix with homemade chocolate icing, so technically, *not* a chocolate cake. We have differing opinions on what we prefer in virtually everything else. Maybe that's a bit of an exaggeration, but not much. With effort, we have prioritized balance in our diet through some specific strategies. Our process is not carved in stone, and we tweak it periodically. Whether you use pieces of our plan or develop your own, be sure to tailor it to your family's needs. As in our family, your needs will change as your schedules, health needs, and living situations evolve. Besides our busy schedule, we must pay attention to diet restrictions, the availability of our favorites, changes in preference, and, of course, the ever-present picky eating issue.

Personally, meal planning has become one of my favorite family activities. We use it as our linchpin for teaching preplanning, grocery shopping, cooking, and kitchen cleaning. Competence in all these areas is needed to ensure mealtimes happen with less stress and more success. A bonus is the extended range of life skills your individual gains from these abilities and the conversations that happen as a matter of course. I learn things about the boys, like can the guys look in an index for a recipe, how many ingredients are they sufficiently familiar with to locate in the kitchen or market, and can they complete a shopping list that supports the menu. Involving them from beginning to end reveals the areas where they are able to use life skills without my help, what they have not yet learned, and what we only think they have learned, but clearly have not. We have found that cleaning and organization are among the skills that need improvement. Throughout this journey, I get to spend quality time with my boys. We discuss other important to-do items outside of those that affect meals simply because we are intentionally focusing on what needs to be done and when. I find out which foods are genuinely their favorites and which ones they eat only to humor their dietitian mom. I am perfectly aware I cannot expect them to buy and eat those foods when they live independently someday or go out to a restaurant. Clearly, we still have a lot of work to make those foods part of their repertoire when they cook for themselves, but I am happy we are adding more variety to what they will eat on their own someday and enlarging the skill sets they will need to take care of their meal needs.

Starting Point

The path to building new abilities starts with one step forward from where the current skill level lies. Up-close, personal interactions at mealtime are especially helpful in teaching social competencies and can be a cornerstone to expanding those abilities into adeptness in other situations. I like to start with what is going well. It makes the process more pleasant when we begin by looking at the positives and work toward the negative habits. Analyzing in this order softens the blow of discussing the habits that need be altered. This assessment works for all habits and skills, but let's focus on meals and eating. Undertake this analysis by creating an attitude that encourages personal growth and acceptance of the difficulty involved in acknowledging each person's challenges and points of view. Take it on as a family project, as this is the step where the rubber meets the road, so to speak. Use it as a means for getting everyone working together. We all have social or life skills that need improvement, so keeping that in mind as you support your individual by having the whole family join this process will identify areas where everyone can develop.

    This analysis becomes your roadmap for adding new foods and organizational skills for planning meals, purchasing groceries, and maintaining cleanliness. Write your findings on whatever notetaking medium suits your purpose. You will refer often to your notes and use all of the elements of this exercise in later stories or conversations. For anyone who thinks nothing related to mealtimes is going well, think about what each person communicates when resistant to new experiences. If your meals are frustrating and challenging, identifying skills everyone already does well may take a bit of thought. Let's face it, most of us did not learn to compliment others during challenging or stressful activities. We tend to point out the things that bother us, but with some thought, there should be a few positives on the list for everyone who participates in meals with your individual. Here are a few possibilities someone might be doing well to help you get started:

- Eating specific foods
- Sharing about their day
- Ability to use utensils, cups, etc.
- Setting the plates and flatware on the table
- Using their napkin
- Chewing with their mouth closed
- Identifying when they feel full

- Having something positive to say
- Sitting in their chair for (insert time)
- Allowing others at the table to eat foods they, personally, do not like
- Finding a reason to smile
- Keeping the family on schedule
- Demonstrating what they have learned during meals
- Helping with clean-up

As you look through this list, you may find none of these skills are yet where you want them to be, but you hopefully will find some area where basic abilities exist. List those; they are the point from which you want to build.

Teaching Opportunities

As you begin, remember the success of this method depends on edifying each other. With that in mind, one of the opportunities taking meals together presents is learning how to competently handle mistakes in a positive manner that does not make your individual feel overwhelmed. While none of us enjoy discussing our missteps in life, it is helpful to our individuals to hear how others are affected by our errors. In our family, we are currently working on acknowledging mistakes, apologizing, and then committing to making a correction. It is vital for everyone to learn that they are not stuck in the same loop every time a situation arises that has caused a previous problem. We can change how we respond, but it does take commitment.

Moving beyond the fixed mindset of believing it's impossible to change because "that's just the way I was made" is essential to reaching goals in all areas of life, whether the individual is working on eating more balanced meals or handling noisy coworkers who make them feel overstimulated and set off anxiety episodes. Believe it or not, deciding to intentionally add vegetables to meals can be a steppingstone to mastering successful ways to deal with rambunctious colleagues.

In fact, meals are a great time for fostering understanding of other's actions. While you are discussing with your individual why they react with fear to a food, you can talk about the events of their day and draw some parallels between your process of understanding their fears and understanding the motivation of someone else's behavior. Maybe the student your individual was annoyed with was being loud because they were overwhelmed with the current situation. Possibly they had not been taught to work quietly and doing so was a new concept to them, or perhaps they had just finished an activity in which they were using a lot of energy and now were having a hard time settling back into a quiet learning environment. Approaching issues from the point of view of trying to understand someone's behavior can change the situational dynamics and provide more options for moving past your individual's frustrations in the same way understanding why your child is having trouble putting a particular food into their mouth can help you work with them as a team to overcome their eating challenges. Involving those with autism in the entire process, start to finish, develops the skills they need in order to be autonomous. Many adults who have autism do not have these necessary skills. Some challenges I see in adults with autism are:

- No food shopping experience
- Inability to organize kitchen (food and equipment)

- Fear of cooking
- Fear of textures and untried foods
- Depending on others for meals
- Inability to follow a recipe or cooking instructions
- Lack of knowledge about which foods fit in which nutritional category
- Lack of knowledge about serving sizes
- Lack of knowledge about manners
- Inability to plan a meal
- Unable to eat in the presence of others
- Unable to be with others as they eat
- Unable to work in the same room, like a kitchen, with others
- Consuming only protein bars or protein shakes for nutrition
- Knowledge of how to store leftovers
- Knowledge of how to wash and stack dishes
- Knowledge of properly wiping/cleaning surfaces
- Concept of when a kitchen is completely clean

- Knowledge of ripe vs. unripe vs. overripe fruits and vegetables

Taming the Snack Monster

Before we move into talking about meal planning, let's talk about snacks, as this is an area that can definitely derail your plans. For years Jason carried a peanut butter sandwich with raisins and apple juice, daily. When he was in second grade, it was suggested we allow the use of food as behavioral reinforcers. In his case, the teachers used gummy bears.

While these treats worked for encouraging him to do his schoolwork, the sticky sugar set his teeth up for significant damage. We allowed the use of food reinforcers only for that one year because when I took him to his annual check-up, the pediatrician asked if he were in the process of having dental work done. Though we required him to brush his teeth daily, he did not do it until bedtime. The combination of the gummy bears and raisins throughout the school day stuck to his teeth for an extended time. All these factors snowballed into a major dental event in which he had to be sedated in a hospital to complete all the cavity work. Unfortunately, the decay did not end with the one event once it started. To this date, he is up to $55,000 in dental work.

Generally speaking, snacks easily become a problem. Many people eat just as many or more calories from snacks as they do from meals, but providing extra snacks is not unusual for autism. I understand the motivation that sets this into motion. If you have a child who does not eat at mealtimes or eats very little, when you try to introduce variety, they may refuse to eat even one bite but are still hungry. As parents, in desperation, we frequently offer anything our child will put in their mouth just to ensure they are eating. Not only have I been tempted to feed my own child snacks, but in the course of my work as a consulting dietitian, I have had parents tell me their child would eat no food at all during meals, but in the course of my visit, they fed the child more calories in snacks than they probably would have received in a meal. My solution to this conundrum is counting the snacks. I encourage using a chart to do this. Determine how many snacks are acceptable in one day and how many fruits or vegetables versus other snack items you want the child to eat. Create a chart with the appropriate daily snacks; then consult the chart when the individual asks for a snack. If the chart shows there are no snacks left for the day, it is the chart's fault, not yours nor that of any family member. Making the chart the "bad guy" in this situation deflects blame from others.

We also predetermine serving sizes for snacks to avoid conflict. A serving of cookies is three small ones. A pudding serving is one small container or a ramekin when we make it ourselves. A serving of cake is a slice one-inch thick, if it is a round cake, or three inches by three inches, if it is rectangular.

Everyone gets one serving of snacks daily as adults, but I allowed two when the boys were children. Everyone at my house follows the same rules. Your rules do not have to be precisely the same but decide what they are, and if you need them, make a chart for the refrigerator and mark off a snack for each one eaten.

Lemons Food Project to the Rescue!

When the boys were in high school, I decided to add more variety to our diet. I had this grand idea of doing something I called *Gourmet Night*. I would make a complete meal using recipes nobody in the family had ever tried. There was always an entree, a non-starchy vegetable, a starch, and a dessert. While I planned to do this once a month, I quickly discovered that a venture of this size took me all day to carry out, so it happened much less often in reality. Surprisingly, the meals were more successful than I had hoped. With everything on the table being something nobody had previously eaten, everyone was more willing to try it. No one was required to eat anything they did not like, and if it was offensive enough, they could quietly spit it into a napkin and immediately dispose of it. From there, we compared those foods to other new foods. I would use similarity to increase acceptance by pointing out something like a vegetable they had liked on *Gourmet Night* had the same spices as this new vegetable. Or maybe I would say, "Remember that meat you liked on Gourmet Night? This meat has the same vinegar on it as the meat you liked." Now, we will all try any new food once.

Today, Gourmet Night has morphed into the *Lemons Food Project*. I prepare something not typically eaten a different way each week for a month. Everyone shares their opinions, and they know I usually post them on social media. I won't say it is their favorite activity, but they have come to tolerate it well and feel they are helping others. I don't allow eating a peanut butter sandwich instead, and I don't allow criticism or negative comments about anyone's choices. However, I did make an exception to this rule when we were trying beets prepared in various ways as our food for the month, and it was *not* going well. I bought some beet chips and then roasted beets in the oven the following week. Jason did not like them at all. He looked over at me during the roasted beet's trial and said, "I'm not feeling the beet, Mom." Did someone tell you people with autism don't have a sense of humor? Well, they are wrong. We stopped the beet trials at two weeks instead of the usual four.

Be Positive!

It may go without saying, but the conversation should always stay positive. If one of the adults at the table makes a face or indicates they do not like the new food, the child/individual will be much less likely to try it. Lemons Food Project is part of this strategy for my family. We have had some hits and some misses, like beet night, but everyone, including these two somewhat picky parents, has been more willing to try new foods if we all participate. One of my family agreements is that I will not hide an ingredient that is not currently accepted inside an accepted food without telling them. For example, I wouldn't hide onions in a casserole, if my children did not like onions and weren't aware I was going to do that. We have this agreement for two reasons. First, I want them to learn to eat foods without having to hide them, especially when served in a public situation like a social gathering. Second, it preserves trust, which is all important. These ground rules help everyone feel more at ease at mealtimes.

Lemons Family Dinner Ground Rules

1. No substitute foods. We do not short-order cook.
2. Conversation about food will stay positive.
3. All efforts will be encouraged.
4. Trying new foods is always celebrated. "Trying" includes cutting a food or mashing with a fork, picking it up and smelling it, or licking it.
5. Meals will include at least two foods each person likes.
6. I will not hide unacceptable foods in acceptable foods.
7. Meals are eaten only at the table.
8. Nobody is required to sit at the table for more than 20 minutes.
9. When meals are over, eating is done.
10. Everyone is encouraged to talk about daily challenges during the meal.
11. Everyone will take part in either cooking, cleaning, or food storage before leaving the kitchen.
12. We will not try too many goals at once.

If I had to name any strategy as being the one that made the biggest difference in reducing stress at mealtime and being the one that helped us increase the variety of food more than any other strategy, it would be developing trust. If your life only has space to add one goal, I recommend implementing the tactics described in this chapter. When we started working on improving trust, I expected it would make meals more pleasant, though I had my doubts about increasing the variety of foods we all ate. But to my surprise, feeling safe enough to say, "I don't like that," has genuinely given everyone permission to not only dislike a food but also to like new foods. We enjoy the open conversation about whether it is perfect or if we would make it differently the next time. Most of the time, we have suggestions to incorporate the next time it is prepared. Preparing and eating new foods has become a fun adventure for our family that has brought us together in new ways.

Our Journey

Over time, we have prioritized our mealtime to foster optimal health and strong relationships with those we hold close. The *Lemons Food Project* has been wonderful for being intentional about incorporating an ever-increasing food variety in general, especially a larger repertoire of vegetables, and periodically even some desserts. Planning which foods we will eat throughout the week is a family affair and has brought us together. Everyone is encouraged to participate, from menu suggestions to shopping, preparing, eating, and all the way to cleaning up. We have not perfected our process, but then, we aren't perfect people. We don't attempt to include all the food groups (proteins, grains, fruits, vegetables, and dairy) in every regular meal. Most days we strive for three, saving the extra work involved with using all food groups for special occasions when we gather with friends or family. To get us started, we use the MyPlate graphic below to help us plan, but we have modified it for our purposes. The graphic is available for download at the URL below the figure. Initially, in the space for each food group, I typed the foods our family would eat. Planning our meals with two foods each person likes is not as easy as it sounds because it's unlikely everyone enjoys the same two foods. While one of us may like only the protein and carbohydrates portions, another may prefer the protein and vegetables. Fortunately, we enjoy enough variety to be able to ensure everyone likes the protein presented and we have at least one side dish on the table that everyone agrees on. That way when we try new recipes, no one leaves the table hungry. As I mentioned in the previous chapter, we attempt to add foods to our list one gently scaffolded step at a time.

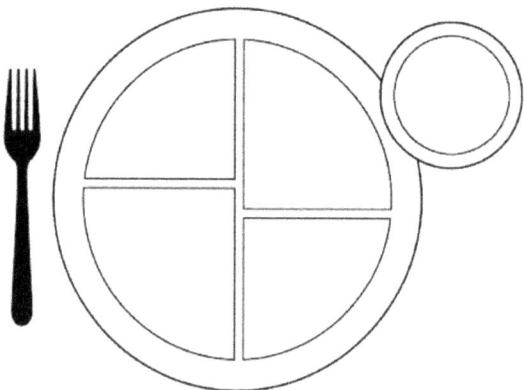

Figure 4-1
Create Your Own MyPlate Menu.pdf (aureedge.us)
https://myplate-prod.azureedge.us/sites/default/files/2020-12/Create%20Your%20Own%20MyPlate%20Menu.pdf

Making it Work for the Long Term

Though we use the food groups found on MyPlate, I'm happy to say that our list has grown so much it no longer fits on the graphic, so I now have a separate list of accepted foods. But as you can see in the graphic below, we started with very few choices, some of which were cooked differently than we eat them now. Carrots and dairy products were particularly challenging. Some of us like raw carrots, while others prefer steamed, not boiled. Jason has not drunk milk since he was eighteen months old, but he will eat his weight in yogurt, especially blueberry yogurt. We will all eat cheese, but Richard will not eat a piece of cheese, like a cheese stick, so his needs to be grated, melted or sliced. While these sensory preferences can make it challenging, they are not insurmountable.

Most of the time, for breakfast my guys eat something from each of these categories: dairy, fruits, and grains. Lunch is a protein and a grain, but sometimes we will meet our three-food group goal with fruit or dairy added.

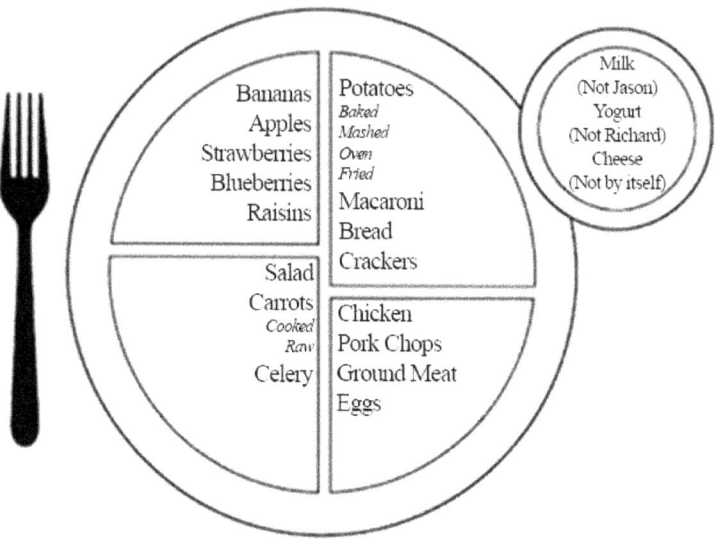

Figure 4-2
Create Your Own MyPlate Menu.pdf (aureedge.us)
https://myplate-prod.azureedge.us/sites/default/files/2020-12/Create%20Your%20Own%20MyPlate%20Menu.pdf

Note: Info typed on the plate is our family's food preferences. Only the plate can be found on MyPlate.

As always, meal planning and even food grouping has to be tailored to the specific health needs of your family. As I stated earlier, one of our basic rules is to have food from three different food groups at each meal, but I have modified MyPlate in our house just a bit because I have diabetes. The grains category includes all starchy, high-carb foods, so mashed potatoes and other high carbohydrate vegetables go in the grains category, as shown in Fig. 4-2. Therefore, our vegetable category consists solely of those items that are lower in carbohydrates. We may also use fruit in place of another starchy food. The method we are working towards is the traditional Diabetes Plate Method recommendation, which fills half the plate with non-starchy vegetables, but we realize we need to increase the number of vegetables everyone eats before that can become a reality. Information on the Diabetes Plate Method can be found at <u>What is the Diabetes Plate Method? (diabetesfoodhub.org)</u>.

With a higher incidence of diabetes in the autism population, I encourage others to do the same, preventively. Having to change the types of foods allowed in each category is confusing after someone gets a diagnosis like pre-diabetes or diabetes. Receiving one of these diagnoses is overwhelming and scary enough without having to unlearn all you ever knew about meal planning. To sum up our strategy, we combine the Diabetes Plate Method with MyPlate. Both are established meal planning tools we use to fit our needs instead of allowing either method's constraints to overwhelm us.

A Word about Sweets and Serving Sizes

Periodically, sweets are part of our meals. Sometimes our desserts are made with artificial sweeteners, but not always. In either case, we talk about serving sizes. Remember that cake serving size I mentioned in the section called *Taming the Snack Monster*? I started this practice when we were at an extended family member's home for dinner, and I looked up to see one of our guys had decided he wanted some cake, so he served himself CAKE – enough for four people! Since this was at a relative's home, and he had yet to take a bite, we took the cake back, cut off a more appropriate serving size, and changed our plan for approaching sweets. Along the way, I have realized conversations about absolutely everything are appropriate for autism. If you want them to learn your idea of manners or your philosophy on health, then you need to verbally express your thoughts and have your individual repeat them back to you. You can have them restate the concepts by saying, can I check to make sure you understood what I said? Please tell me what we just discussed to ensure I was clear.

Our Planning Process

We begin our meal planning with the one meal where we know we will all sit down together, the evening meal, which we write on our planning calendar. We start with the protein, or entree portion, of the meal, which I do for a couple of reasons. First, we tend to agree more frequently on protein choices. Second, we have been specifically working on variety with this portion. Since we have already set a precedent with previous meals, we choose what we want for the protein and then discuss how to prepare it. Our typical choices are ground meat, chicken, turkey, fish, or pork. Plant-based proteins work for this portion, as well. As we are planning, we try to recognize the days when we will have too much on our schedule to be able to pull off a home-cooked meal and notate it on the schedule. If your individual enjoys eating out, it gives them something to look forward to; if they dread eating out, you can prepare them in advance for the event. Placing it in your calendar allows you to discuss strategies for coping with whatever is overwhelming.

When we add our protein to the menu, we make sure we do not repeat the same kind of food more than every three days, so that a typical week might start with chicken on Sunday, pork chops on Monday, and tacos on Tuesday. After planning our protein for the week, we add in carbs. Typical choices include foods made from potatoes, beans, or pasta. Lastly, we add our non-starchy vegetables. Candidly, I can tell you this is the one choice that changes most frequently, simply because while one of our mainstays is a salad, if the lettuce has any brown at all, it is a no-go.

After we have completed the evening meal planning, we generally work on our grocery list, keeping in mind what we need for our breakfast, lunch, and snack lists. Breakfast for us stays routine. I would like to encourage three food groups at breakfast, but I am also realistic enough to cut everyone slack. Not one of us is a morning person, so we settle for two, easy food groups. It seems to help us all get out the door more efficiently, as following the same routine in the morning means we are more likely to make it to the car with everything we need. Any change in habit can throw the other habits out of sync.

Tip: Because my life tends to be more hectic than I'd like, as a backup, I count how many items I am supposed to have with me when I walk out the door (Three bags – lunch, computer, purse and three other items – keys, phones, and nametag).

As we make our grocery lists, sometimes using a meal planning app, sometimes a spreadsheet, and sometimes using old-fashioned pen and paper, depending on what skill I am currently working on with my boys, we practice taking inventory of the food we have on hand and whether it is fresh and safe to eat. Checking for availability and freshness is a self-sufficiency responsibility that needs to be learned by everyone in the house. Therefore, we rearrange our menu to use food while it is fresh, as we check dates. Teaching your individual to discard food regularly to prevent food-borne illness will help ensure healthy, lifelong habits when you are no longer assisting with their food preparation. I have everyone in the family read freshness dates, and in the process, I have learned I also needed to teach the difference between a "use by" date and a "best by" date. This practice is a cornerstone to keeping the pantry and refrigerator free of what we refer to as science projects, our term for moldy food. Writing the date on the individual packages of the food before refrigerating or freezing is helpful, especially since we often make the same recipes. Is that leftover taco meat mom intends to use in a salad from this Tuesday or last Tuesday? The only way to know for sure is to date it.

In reviewing our grocery items, we can quickly see where there is a task needed to follow through on the list: a run to the store to purchase ingredients, food moved from the freezer to the refrigerator to be thawed, or maybe we find that a completely different meal should be prepared. Sometimes we have had to phone our sons to have them start a meal because we have been delayed, and other times we have needed a quick substitution. For example, recently, this was due to an approaching storm that was expected to cause power outages.

Because everyone is responsible for their own breakfast and

lunch, reviewing food items we have on hand helps plan for those meals. Our sons have jobs and can buy their food and snacks when they are not home, so we make sure to discuss which foods we need to add to the grocery list to complete our meals and which foods they will buy outside of home meals. If these talks reveal a nutritional pattern I find concerning, such as too many unhealthy snacks or quick meals, we talk about why it's a concern and how to replace it with a habit that supports their goals. I would love to say we have perfected our process and never change a menu at the last minute, but that is not true. When we notice certain foods showing up too frequently in our meals over a week or month, we work on changing habits by discussing how often we should repeat favorite foods. As is common with anyone, telling my sons that a food is not allowed, only makes them want it even more. So, we talk about making positive choices that *do* **fit** into our meal plan instead of focusing on eliminating those that *don't*. The only problem food in our house is corn, as one of my sons is allergic to it. That said, while most of our meals are corn-free, we do use some recipes that include corn. This creates an opportunity to practice the life skill of reading ingredient lists and avoiding foods you cannot eat. We set up our calendar using predictable patterns, making changes easy to accomplish. These patterns allow us to slip in a different food from the same nutritional group when we discover a particular food will not work, whether due to unavailability or some other reason.

After each evening meal, during clean-up, we review the modified MyPlate chart as our basis and check the ingredients for the next day's evening meal to make sure we have not overlooked anything. The one thing most likely to send us to a restaurant is neglecting to thaw menu items, so we make checking frozen items our starting point, then look for all the other ingredients to determine where we might need to make substitutions. Scaffolding in one routine at a time as we check to make sure we have everything for the next day, we add foods to our grocery list for the following week and complete our end of the day cleaning.

Keep in mind as you customize these strategies for your own

family that it is key to remember the importance of challenging only one skill at a time. Our sons are adults, and this journey has been long. We have learned through trial and error, and while some of the skills and planning methods I discuss may sound advanced, in the beginning, I assure you they were not. You will see me state this often because it matters: you always have to begin where the individual is currently. Meal planning does not need to be complicated or original each time; many people eat the same combination of foods regularly. Using a consistent combination of foods for meals can make it easier for families and can be a springboard for expanding variety by merging components from other accepted meals.

Cooking from recipes everyone is familiar with makes developing our grocery list predictable. Most of our recipes are committed to memory. We verbally review the menu and the items needed to complete the grocery list. We pull out written recipes to ensure we have everything on our list as a double-check at the end of our grocery planning. A helpful addition to your menu planning system might be a written list of grocery items. Remember, this facilitates learning, so have your individual involved. They need to learn every part of the process. One week they might write the list or enter it into the app, then the next week, they could be asked to check which ingredients are already on hand. To confirm they have learned all the process pieces, have them do the task without you, then verify they did not miss anything. You won't realize how much support you are giving until you pull yourself out of the process.

I was surprised that my sons, who had prepared recipes side-by-side with me regularly, could not complete them when I walked out of the kitchen. Adding an ingredient someone hands you is a different skill set than finding and measuring that ingredient yourself to add to a recipe. You won't know if your individual possesses the ability to accomplish such tasks without your being present in the room until you try it out. I learned I needed to prepare a recipe with them, have one of the boys add an ingredient to the recipe when I walked out of the room, and then work on them completing the recipe without me being present. Each step is a growth process. Unknowingly, I gave them cues in ways I never thought about when I was present. It takes multiple times of practicing skills for anyone to feel confident, but a person with autism usually needs more practice than their peers.

They also need to be allowed to make mistakes. When mistakes happen, you learn which skills to work on next and where knowledge gaps exist. Like everyone else, they learn more from mistakes than from doing things correctly but may need someone to help with identifying the necessary corrections.

During the process of allowing the boys to practice some kitchen skills on their own, I recently discovered that one of my sons did not know how to find information in an index by looking for a recipe in alphabetical order. It suddenly made sense to me why he could not find spices I had in alphabetical order and never put them back in the same place.

The menu plan shown in Figure 4.3 is a guide we use to lead us through the meal planning process and cooking, and you may find it helpful. This graphic makes last minute changes easier. Because of the recipe's inclusion, these meal sheets can become a printed recipe book to save time and to have for when your individual moves to a different living situation at some point in their life.

Meal Planning Sheet

Menu

Entrée:
Ingredients needed:
1. _____
2. _____
3. _____
4. _____
5. _____
6. _____

Entrée Cooking Instructions

Time to prepare entree recipe:
Start preparing at:

Starch:
Ingredients needed:
1. _____
2. _____
3. _____
4. _____
5. _____
6. _____

Starch Cooking Instructions

Time to prepare starch recipe:
Start preparing at:

Vegetable:
Ingredients needed:
1. _____
2. _____
3. _____
4. _____
5. _____
6. _____

Vegetable Cooking Instructions

Time to prepare vegetable recipe:
Start preparing at:

Figure 4-3
James Lemons, III©

Mealtime Management

One of my sons and I set alarms on our phones to remind us to start cooking so dinner will not be late. For recipes that take longer than forty-five minutes, we schedule time on the weekend to do prep work in advance. We are by no means always successful at getting meals done early enough, though we usually do not have to rush to finish everything before bedtime, but our efforts in improving time management have helped. We have also learned to experiment mainly on weekends with recipes that make us curious – recipes similar to what we already like with the ingredients changed just a little are some of our favorites. Some of these may even feature a different main ingredient but have similar flavors to a dish we already like. We are generally ready to do something easy on Friday, and Sunday is often full of family activities. Incorporating our predicted energy levels on busier days of the week and taking into consideration other time commitments like exercise, scheduled pet care, and trash days also helps keep us on track. We try to schedule our meals on days with fewer time-consuming tasks competing for our attention. Limiting the work-intensive meals to days when we have more time available teaches lessons about having appropriate boundaries that reduce stress.

Making it Work for You

If your family eats three vegetables, two proteins, and five starches, start with those. Combine these foods in as many ways as possible, but be aware that altering preferred combinations may be your first challenge. It is not unusual for me to discover that individuals always eat one food with another specific food. One way to increase meal variety is to add one extra item to an accepted combination. Chicken nuggets are often considered the unofficial national food of autism, so let's use them for our example. If your individual eats only French fries with their nuggets, start by adding another food to the plate, like carrot sticks, for example. If your individual needs their food to be a specific texture, maybe whole or broken into ten pieces, writing not only new foods, but a new texture, into the prominently displayed menu is an excellent place to start preparing your individual for change. It gives them time to process what is coming and develops their trust that you will let them know of alterations in advance. A whiteboard or chalkboard can serve the purpose of displaying the menu of the day. Your system needs to be one that works for you and your individual. While I use an actual whiteboard calendar, there are several options, including:

- Printed calendar
- Menu Cards or sheets, such as Figure 4.3
- Bullet Planners
- Spreadsheets
- MyPlate graphics with the meal written on it
- Binder with tabs for meals and the recipes that go with them

To help your individual overcome the challenge of newness once you are at the table, it often helps to have someone the individual admires and trusts model enjoying the change. Have them add the carrot sticks to their plate and comment positively about them. If your individual eats their chicken nuggets whole, have the person assisting you in the exercise say something like,

"I think I want to have half nuggets, today," as they cut them in front of the individual.

The Starting Point

Develop your system with the food your family agrees on the most as the cornerstone. Obviously, building trust and reducing stress for the entire family is a major goal. For our purposes and simplicity's sake, let's use those chicken nuggets again for this example. During this time, your individual may eat chicken nuggets for a while, build trust, and then progress to other challenges as everyone builds a comfort level. Write their chicken nuggets on the menu for the individual but plan other foods for the family. Encourage them to place the other foods on their plate in tiny amounts without pressure to eat them. As other family members thoroughly, obviously, enjoy their food, encourage the individual to try smelling, ripping, smashing, and checking out every sensory aspect of the food while you watch for cues that they might be ready to bring it close to their face.

Family members get bonus points to demonstrate how much they like those foods and enjoy themselves at the table while maintaining table manners. Exaggerated enjoyment of food is a plus, as long as the individual does not react negatively to the exaggeration. *Everything* should be person-centered. If they respond to exaggeration, go for it. If they are upset by exaggeration, leave the dramatics off. This process will develop habits. Mealtime discussion should include sharing your appreciation of a sibling or other tablemate who tried a new food or an accepted food prepared in a new recipe. Point out behaviors of those at the table which you would like to see repeated, like wiping their face or cutting up their food in small portions. If you ever say to the individual, "Don't do [that]," whatever [that] is should be put on your list of practice items and becomes a candidate for a story. As the saying goes, which dog will become the strongest? The one you feed. In the same way, the behavior or habit you want to become the strongest is the one that deserves the most discussion.

Adding New Foods

We added new items into our meal plan by starting with foods we already enjoyed, as seen in the MyPlate graphic previously. Using a person-centered approach when considering which challenge to take on next, we took on the one we felt was most important to us or the one causing the most distress for one of the family members. It is essential to increase both the variety and number of foods individuals with autism will eat for many reasons, but starting at the individual's current comfort level and ability is critical. Creating a healthy, calm atmosphere for everyone to come together is the top priority, then you can add food. Nobody's eating routine stays permanently set, nor should it. One of the frustrations I have witnessed for some families has involved food changes that are entirely out of their control. Even a color change in the packaging of a favorite food can cause a meltdown. I know that from personal experience, but more about that in a later chapter. As time goes by, changes in health or lab values requiring intervention make it necessary to increase, decrease, or eliminate foods from our eating routine.

Preestablished habits of giving new foods a try makes this process easier.

Increasing Acceptance

Once meals have become a comfortable, joyful experience where trust is part of the equation, it is time to start increasing the number of foods your individual will eat. By taking a growth-mindset approach, if you can add one new item to the accepted foods list per month, you will have tried twelve new foods by the end of the year. Twelve new foods may be four times as many as your individual was eating than when you first started trying to expand your diet.

So how do you add new foods? I do this in a couple of ways. While occasionally I start the process by seeing a recipe from Pinterest or maybe in the family recipe box, I also like to start by choosing three different foods for everyone to vote on. We discuss unique ways to fix the same food. My goal is to prepare it in four completely different recipes. However, many foods have several varieties. For instance, we may try different types of lettuce, apples, pickles, or cookies. Our most significant rule is that the food needs to be new to everyone. At this point, everyone will take a bite. Rarely is anyone unable to chew up one bite and swallow it, but everyone knows they will not have to take a second bite if they did not like the first.

We often have to make changes to our menu, but that allows us to help the boys build skills to deal with changes in other areas of their lives. It is all just part of the process. In fact, dealing with unexpected changes in all areas of life is a significant challenge for many individuals who have autism. While my family now eats every evening together at the table, I acknowledge this is not how many families eat. Honestly, we did not always eat all meals at the table when our children were younger. Families have many obligations and outside interests. When the family is not eating at the table, acknowledge and talk about it using a story or frank discussion. We build this into our calendar, as well. Handling plans, changes and challenges at home as a family has allowed us to do some of the work without public meltdowns. Even if you are not eating at a table together daily, carve out and spend some time together. You will be pleasantly surprised by the benefits.

Creating Your Own Framework

Each task needed to cook meals then clean a kitchen needs to be reviewed for understanding. Our sons either seem to become compulsive about every little task or have no idea they need to complete various tasks. I find using a checklist helpful, but it does not have to be a written list. Using needed items as a visual list is impactful and, often, more memorable. Pictures can be an essential part of teaching the skills. Many resources already exist with recipes that include images of all the ingredients and tools needed, as well as accurately measured ingredients. These are great assets. I also encourage you to make some of these for yourself. Nothing works as well as having photos of the same items you use at home, and cell phones make this easy. The differences between stock photos of yellow measuring cups and photos of my own green Tupperware measuring cups could be confusing to my boys. My future goals include having a website with many recipes that users can customize by uploading photos of their own tools and ingredients. This is on my to-do list, but it's a long list. In the meantime, if you want to take this idea and run with it, go for it!

For your individual to gain independent cooking skills, choosing recipes with clear instructions is imperative. You may use the "recipe" Grandma scribbled on a napkin, which in reality, is just a list of ingredients with measurements like pinch and dash, but for your individual, you'll need to rewrite the instructions to include all steps in an organized manner with specific measurements. I have included a standard recipe format below. Each recipe should include a grocery list and the time needed to complete each stage. Individuals with autism tend to believe activities take no time. No time means zero seconds, so they always seem to be scrambling to catch up or have meltdowns when it is time to move on to the next task.

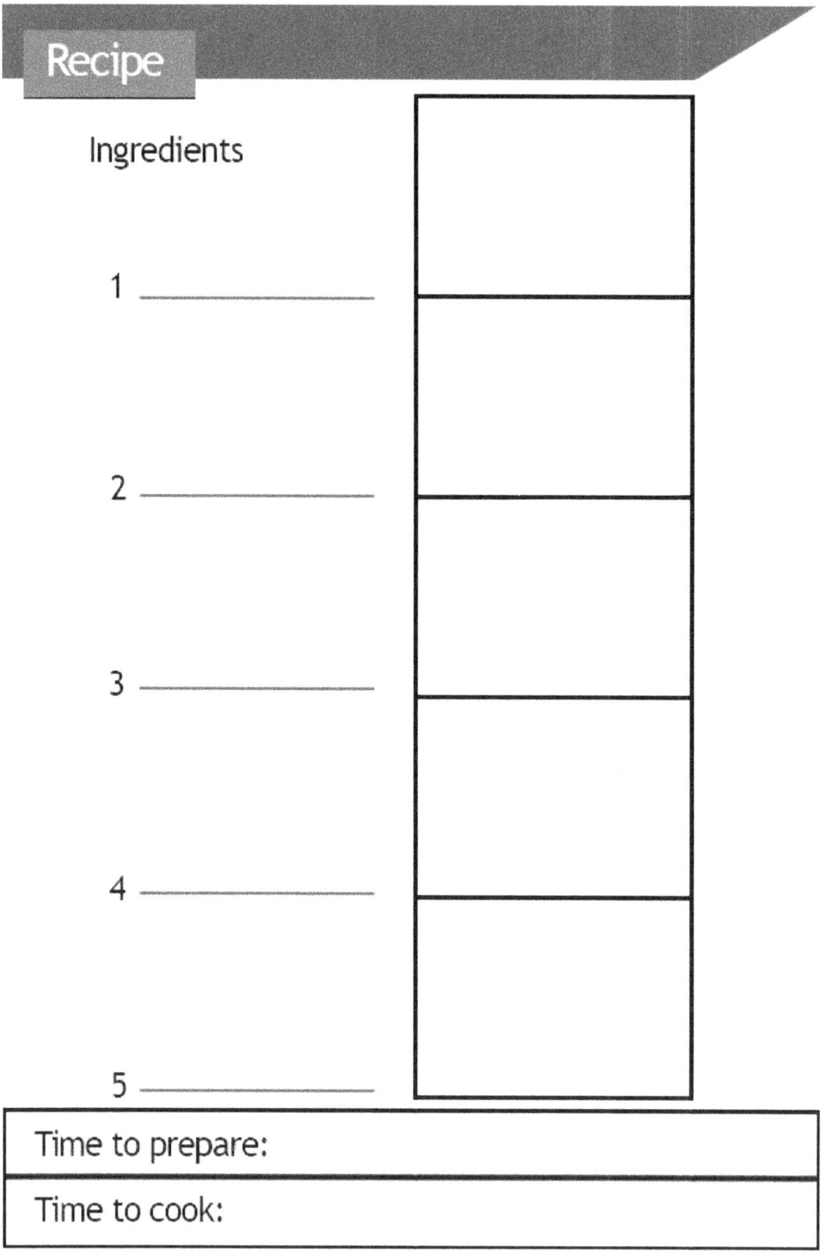

Recipe

Ingredients

1 _____

2 _____

3 _____

4 _____

5 _____

Time to prepare:
Time to cook:

Figure 4-4
James Lemons, III©

Recipe

Instructions

1 _____

2 _____

3 _____

4 _____

5 _____

| Time to prepare: |
| Time to cook: |

Figure 4-5
James Lemons, III©

Contingency meals

As you develop your menu system, remember to create at least one "in-a-hurry meal." Preplanning allows for those days when things just aren't going right. No matter how much we plan, there will be times when circumstances get in the way. That is typical for life, but our individuals with autism do not tend to handle those times well, and it is challenging to think through how to make things calm and consistent for our individuals in the middle of the unexpected. Having that go-to backup plan to pull out can smooth the way. Examples of "in-a-hurry meals" include:

- Prepared heat-and-eat meals
- Meals that require no cooking
- Food that can be eaten on the move
- Foods that can be handed off to an alternate caregiver

Food Prep and Kitchen Skills

As in developing many skills, children should be involved in the preparation of daily meals. This might mean putting sliced potatoes in a bowl so you can pour them into a hot pan of water or using a lettuce knife to cut salad. The task should be developmentally appropriate and take into consideration how far along in their sensory journey your individual is, but the more they are with the sights, sounds, textures, and smells of cooking, the easier this process will be. Food preparation is an excellent place to start addressing sensory challenges, especially since there is no expectation of putting the food in one's mouth during the cooking stage. The tasks will vary according to their progress through the developmental stages, but some age-appropriate kitchen tasks include:

- Handing dishes to be placed in the dishwasher
- Setting the table
- Cutting/Tearing lettuce
- Washing fresh produce
- Peeling potatoes

- Spreading (peanut butter, jelly, butter, mayonnaise, etc.)
- Making name cards for seating assignments
- Taking out the trash
- Sweeping the floor

Many I talk to have intense fears of the stove, so I encourage teaching stove safety. Can your child stir a pot or turn the grilled cheese when old enough? Are they able to use a potholder or glove to move an item from one point to another on the cabinet and then safely move an item from the stove? Can this be accomplished using a hand-over-hand method? Teaching cooking skills using crock pots, electric skillets, microwaves, or other less intimidating appliances may be appropriate. Community Support Systems in Maryland has a very helpful website with recipes designed for those learning cooking skills, which can be found at [Community Support Services (css-md.org)](https://css-md.org).

Often our individuals have felt stress surrounding mealtimes, specifically in the kitchen. If tensions have been too high in the kitchen previously, their journey may need to start by preparing foods in another area, like mixing tuna salad in the living room on a TV tray. Starting this journey may involve counseling for your individual, you, or both. Take your cues from the individual to determine what support they need to take the next step, then move forward as a team.

Eating Away from Home

Everyone will have occasions to eat somewhere outside their home; therefore, it is also important to discuss expectations and appropriate manners when eating at other places, especially if your child will be filling their own plate. We talk with our boys about what we expect them to put on their plates. The food they serve themselves may be something they previously put together at home, or, if someone else is serving portions, we may discuss polite ways to say, "I am just not hungry right now; I'll eat later." Something along the lines of "I'll have this granola bar, but thank you anyway," is also acceptable. Allowing your individual to bring a different food option may require alerting the host before arrival, so they are not taken by surprise. While discussing your individual's mealtime needs with the host may be uncomfortable or stressful, it will help prevent an awkward situation for your individual. Remember, for some, the step of being with others while they eat – even if it is something they are accustomed to eating in the presence of others – may be a great deal of progress, but if more than one skill is challenged, it may become more than is bearable. As there is a progression in skill sets, they should eventually learn how to have those conversations themselves and ask for reasonable accommodation at restaurants.

Additionally, eating meals with others outside the immediate family is an effective way for children to learn social skills while their parents can be present to guide them. Mealtimes with others someplace besides our home, especially in someone else's home, is also where I learn how much I am inadvertently facilitating situations for the guys with those around them. I like to watch and listen to their interactions quietly. At these times, I learn where we need to work on manners, what we need to discuss about serving ourselves at the home of others, and what we need to discuss about boundaries.

Typical discussions following one of these meals include:

- Please put at least three foods on your plate.
- If you put just a few beans on your plate, that tells your host immediately you are not happy with your choice and are being forced to eat this by some unseen force. Please put a serving that indicates this is a food you might like to eat.
- Please look around and see how many people are present. If you take so much food that others will not be able to have an equal serving, that isn't polite. Real life example: Huge pieces of cake!
- Please take *and* use a napkin. Either look at people when they are talking or join the conversation. (Note: I recognize that looking at someone, talking to them, and hearing what they say is difficult for someone with autism. If this is the case, please tell others you are listening to them but it is easier for you if you look at your plate instead of their face.)

Meals with others is a good time for me to enjoy my position as a fly on the wall, make my mental list of what we need to work on next, and celebrate our successes. It is always good to hear the boys having conversations and watch them prove they really have learned all those lessons about manners while eating at other places. I also hear when others lead them easily. Since I want to develop the skill of keeping good boundaries and resisting when others might lead them into trouble, we discuss how it is okay to have your own feelings and opinions and decline to participate in conversations and activities that might be hurtful to yourself or others.

Finishing Up

Mealtime isn't truly complete until everything is cleaned up afterward. We incorporate routines for cleaning up and, in the process, teach skills that can be incorporated elsewhere. Bringing the dishes to the sink or the dishwasher, accompanied by conversations about being responsible for cleaning up after yourself, can be applied to any cleaning task in the home. This conversation can happen in a couple of ways. The inverse conversation may be appropriate as you teach the importance of keeping a clean area to reduce germs and make the living space more pleasant. Many individuals with autism have sensory issues with anything out of place or messy, like sticky foods on their hands. However, they often do not know *how* to prevent the mess. Letting them know it is okay and can be cleaned with little work may help reduce their anxiety. The phrase "it's okay, things happen and we can clean it up" may be important for reducing the anxiety caused by having a mess in the first place. Both of my sons clean at this point, but I saw this phrase in action when, to my amazement, my son most likely upset with spills or disorder suddenly said, "It's okay, things happen; we can clean it up." He did not get that mantra from me. He learned it at work, where his supervisor used it with him. That one phrase has been truly helpful in getting past his frustrations, whether it was a spill, something broken, or something that did not go as planned. We have learned to be grateful when someone else teaches our sons new things.

Your idea of a clean kitchen and that of your child's will invariably be a different vision, so here's a word of advice: Be obvious about your goals and expectations. It's important to remember that individuals with autism are not good at picking up inferences. If I say, "The trash sure is getting full," my sons are likely to acknowledge this is true and go about their day. They don't understand that was a hint they should take out the trash. The best practice is to say what you want. Typically, they won't learn something just by watching you because it is too easy to misinterpret what they see. I have noticed that I am quicker to add a conversation to our discussion list when I get embarrassed in public. Usually, this tells me I have not paid enough attention to what the boys were trying to tell me with their behaviors. As a visual help, I set out all the tools needed, and put them away as we finish using them. My inspiration for using items rather than a written list comes from the TEACCH program (Mesibov, 2005). It took a while to realize that incorporating predictability is one of the best methods for getting through the day. The TEACCH Program has used a system of charts or objects placed in a specific order to create a predictable flow of activities from their onset.

Our clean-up checklist has evolved over time and includes:

- Clear and clean table
- Wash dishes (dishwasher or by hand)
- Clear and clean countertops
- Clean stove top
- Wipe sink
- Check trash to determine if it needs to be carried out

(Note: We clean our floors using robot vacuums; therefore, it is not part of our daily after-meal routine, but you may find it helpful to include in yours.)

You may want to have a more thorough checklist as you start this journey, so I have included a comprehensive one in the appendix for your convenience.

Not only do individuals with autism not interpret hints well, transferring a skill they learned in one area to another is not intuitive for them. Intentionally teaching that same or similar skill in a different situation can aid in cementing the knowledge.

Repeated learning opportunities increase the likelihood the individual will be able to transfer the skill to other opportunities on their own eventually. For example, I encourage learning to wash dishes both by hand and by using a dishwasher. Having access to a dishwasher is never guaranteed, and even if you do have one, some day it may break and need repair. Washing by hand is the best way to learn how much pressure you need to exert to scrub away residue, so this skill comes in handy for cleaning bathrooms, cars, and anything else that may need to be scrubbed at some point.

For our family, teaching a broad range of competencies has been a natural and important outgrowth of this process. Like you would build a house foundation on a cornerstone by placing other blocks upon it, we have added other essential abilities such as making lunches for the next day, watering plants, and carrying the trash to the curb.

Our journey has been fluid over time, reflecting the changes of our family dynamics, needs, and personalities. For us, it has not been a trend, but a roadmap to success. In the process, we have broadened our sons' skill sets, bolstered their confidence levels, and replaced fear with curiosity and the enjoyment of trying new foods. Moreover, our need to feel we are doing any and everything to get the guys to eat has been replaced with the joy of pleasant conversations and camaraderie while we eat. Because we have developed a specific strategy for ensuring we have all the ingredients we need and that they are ready to use, we don't eat out nearly as often as we did in the past. When we do eat at restaurants or social gatherings, the habits we have formed at home in supporting each other and being respectful of the individual's needs and preferences translate well into successful meals anywhere. Best of all, our family closeness has been strengthened by this plan, and we feel we are confidently on the path to having our sons be able to have healthy, autonomous lives one day.

Chapter Five

Sensory Explorations

Many individuals with autism have sensory issues that affect eating, but what are sensory issues? Our occupational therapist explained it to me long before anyone was testing for sensory integration therapy needs. Most individuals with autism` are either hyposensitive (not sensitive enough) or hypersensitive (too sensitive), so nowadays, testing is done for mitigation. We use all five senses when we eat, therefore, understandably, someone with sensory issues would have problems at mealtime. On the surface, eating seems very simple, but it is actually a complex process. We expect everyone to sit at the table and politely have conversations. Everyone should eat their food with closed mouths while not reacting negatively to anything on their plate, in the room, or on the table. These will be essential skills to accomplish or find ways to compensate for the lack of them as individuals with autism work towards self-sufficiency. This skill set does not come naturally. Mastering table skills and eating that ever-elusive balanced diet is incredibly challenging for someone who reacts to sensory stimuli during meals.

Bribing or pressuring someone into eating does not result in permanent acceptance or enjoyment of food. In addition, bribery can be costly, as my husband and I learned early on. The animated movie Land Before Time came out when my oldest two sons were five and three. Our eldest, Richard, loved dinosaurs, so this movie was instantly a hit for the boys. One day, we took them to dinner at Wyatt's cafeteria. As we walked through J C Penney to get there, I spotted stuffed dinosaur toys from Land Before Time. I thought there's my hook to get them to eat, so I offered to buy them each a stuffed dinosaur if they would eat *three* bites of mashed potatoes. We thought they would love mashed potatoes if we ever got them just to eat a few bites.

Doesn't everyone? We got our dinner, and the boys worked and worked to get those three bites down.

Richard tended to eat vegetables as though he were taking a pill. He would take a bite, put it in his mouth, then drink water to flush it down. He ate most of his vegetables this way for a long time and, occasionally, still does. On this night, it took him quite a while to accomplish the task of eating three bites of mashed potatoes, but he did it. Jason did not struggle quite as much, but eating those three bites was not easy for him either. Two weary parents took them back to buy their prize only to discover the dinosaurs were Gund stuffed toys and, therefore, expensive. The smallest dinosaur was thirty dollars for one! I had just committed to spending ten dollars for each of the six bites of mashed potatoes, plus the cost of the food. We learned a lot as parents that day. First, this did not end our struggle with mashed potatoes. Jason eventually learned to love mashed potatoes, but his love of potatoes did not happen soon after that incident. It took another few years to get him to that point. Even as an adult, Richard must be reminded not to eat his mashed potatoes like taking medicine. It also taught us to be more aware of what we commit to when we promise a reward for eating a particular food. We have experienced many successes incorporating foods that I would have expected to be more challenging than potatoes. Through it all, and even still, we have used a growth mindset and a mostly stress-free environment to support our sons as they overcome various sensory issues and work through misgivings one step at a time. Rather than the promise of reward, we have moved the pressure to eat foods they may not like, allowing them to use exploration at their own pace.

Acceptance of foods happens incrementally for those who have sensory challenges. As with other skills, learning happens in gradual steps, and only when they feel there will not be any judgment if they back out without taking a bite or decide they don't like it. Previous successes provide a foundation for building future gains. Imagine someone offering you something you were unsure you wanted to eat, like a live octopus. How many steps would it take to put it in your mouth, chew it, swallow it, and possibly even enjoy the experience? Would it be hard to look at and think about eating it? Would the smell bother you? And how much support would you need from those who were with you? Overcoming your misgivings about this new food would not be easy. It would most likely take many tries with various sensory exploration techniques to work towards the possibility of putting it in your mouth. Imagining the experience gives you a glimpse of how complex overcoming sensory challenges is for individuals with this neurodivergence.

Many people would never work past the sensory challenges of eating a live octopus. The good news is that we can have a balanced diet without eating octopuses. Alternate sources of protein or omega-three fatty acids are typically found in seafood and nuts. Foods like chicken, beef, or plant-based alternative meats provide protein. The same is true for your individual's diet. They don't have to eat every single food offered. They are just as entitled to have likes and dislikes as all the rest of us. However, just like everyone else, they need a variety of foods in their diet to ensure growth and good health, so working through challenges to facilitate a diet that sustains good health is essential. We want them to work towards self-sufficiency in maintaining a balanced diet because they have learned to enjoy diverse foods.

Think of our bodies as a car. We know the car does not go unless you put gas in it, but there is more to operating the car than putting fuel in it. Our cars also need all the fluids in the engine to help it operate well and tires with enough tread and air. Now think of the calories we eat as fuel, but like cars, our bodies need more than calories. We need variety that provides protein, carbs, vitamins, and minerals the same way our tires need air or our car's cooling system needs antifreeze. Neglecting any necessary maintenance on our cars will eventually cause a problem. In the same way, if we do not eat enough fiber or vitamins, this will eventually become a health problem.

Progressing through the steps needed for permanent acceptance of foods at the individual's pace, while consistently preserving choice versus compliance, will have a long-term effect on health. The goal should always be balanced meals that support current and future health, which includes the need to work on eating from all food groups. Written goals from feeding therapists often call for increasing foods eaten by a specific number, such as twenty or twenty-five, but this can lead to focusing efforts on one food group only. This never results in a balanced diet, and eventually, this pattern will cause health issues. Therefore, it is essential to increase the nutritional variety, not simply the number of foods, someone will eat. I prefer to use goals that include all food groups; i.e., Susan will eat five foods from each of the four food groups.

Let's look at how the five senses are involved in meals. Remember that individuals with autism have trouble predicting changes and prefer sameness in all areas of their lives, including their meals. Finding ways to cope with these issues requires breaking down obstacles individually and evaluating every piece of their routine. Your role becomes that of investigator. Look carefully at what your individual is doing. This behavior is the tip of the iceberg; what lies underneath that tip is what your child is trying to tell you through their body/behavioral language. In the next section, we will look at some troubleshooting questions to ask yourself as you work to find solutions to your child's specific mealtime challenges.

Looking for Triggers

Start by watching the body language and reactions of everyone at the dinner table then try to answer some of these questions:

Does the stress begin before the meal, during the meal, or towards the close of the meal? Is there a meltdown when they smell the food, after they reach the table, not at all, after the first bite, or at another time? Look at what the individual is doing, not what they are not doing. If you are concerned about their picky eating, it is a given that they are not eating all the foods offered. The clues to where to start are what they do *instead* of eating. If the struggle begins when they get in their chair, you will want to see if they feel steady and supported. Will they sit in their chair without pressure to eat while others eat? Work may need to start with sitting with others during playtime. If they get down to run around as soon as they are placed in the chair, the response is to return to the chair. Straps should be secured, if available, to assist in keeping the child in the chair; if there are no straps, a belt can be used as a seat belt. Alternatively, something like sensory weights or bean bags can be placed in the child's lap.

As you observe, look for consistent reactions. Just like it is difficult to hit a moving target or diagnose a mechanical problem that happens intermittently, it may take several observations to determine why a reaction is happening. It could be to a specific food or even several different foods. It could be that they are anticipating a negative reaction from others to their attempts to eat. Do they eat food that is touching other food? Someone who does not eat food that touches other food may reject casseroles and even mixed foods, like Hamburger Helper, meatloaf, or even cake with icing instead of plain cake. Also, remember that just like the rest of us, the child could be simply having a bad day or not feeling well.

Being objective in the process is not easy. I encourage making a video of a couple of meals, which should be viewed when everyone is rested and calm. Evaluating why meals are challenging is an emotional process, so as you view these videos, commit to making observations instead of accusations. I promise that neither the perfect parent nor the perfect child exists. Work towards solutions. Start your observations with, "While watching the video, I observe [fill in the blank]." Make a list of the observations. Others who know your individual may help make observations; however, I encourage caution when bringing others into this process. Everyone needs to be committed to making unemotional observations and acknowledging those with autism need time to learn skills and adjust to sensory challenges.

Some specific areas to observe include:

- Stability of the seat
- Consistent reactions vs. inconsistent reactions
- Sensory stimuli present or absent
- Environmental conditions that are present (think about the placemat, tablecloth, plate, cup, utensils, and noises in the room)
- Ability to handle the cup or other utensils
- Specific sensory stimuli they seem to enjoy (music, smells, flavors, textures)

- Observe the body language and reactions of everyone at the table and identify clues that set off unwanted behavior.

Feeding Therapy

Another strategy for meeting mealtime challenges head on includes feeding therapy. This practice incorporates exploration and curiosity to expand the accepted textures, flavors, and foods the individual will touch, manipulate, or consume. A professional team working on feeding can be a priceless asset in helping your child to accept new foods. A feeding therapy team should consist of either a speech-language pathologist or occupational therapist, someone trained in counseling like a social worker or professional licensed counselor, and a dietitian. In a perfect world, a feeding team would include all these professionals, but combining even two plus the caregiver and the individual can make a complete team. As I have stated before, the team's lead is the individual, not a therapist or caregiver. It is especially crucial to observe the individual and work with their comfort level when expanding an eating routine to include new foods or new textures of familiar food. As the team works through fears and hesitations, remember nobody likes to be forced to do something, and being forced to eat a food may feel like a physical attack or violation. Consumption of novel foods needs to be entirely voluntary. If you were ever forced to eat a food, it is not likely your favorite now. It may even be a food you will not eat at all. While the team members may encourage, participate, and demonstrate actions they would like to see while maintaining a positive environment, all the tasks should be attainable without hovering. Play during this process can include:

- Stories
- Touching and manipulating food
- Using the food as another object, like a car or train
- Using scents of foods in bubbles (For example, water-soluble items or extracts mixed in with commercial bubble solution.)
- Playdough using foods or spices (Example: Making playdoh recipe that includes canned pumpkin and

pumpkin pie spice. There are many recipes on the internet.)

- Art projects using food

Caregivers should be encouraged to continue food exploration outside of therapy, in their homes. Food exploration does not have to be at every meal, nor should it be. As I have said before, I don't believe every meal should become a therapy session. There is merit to having meals precisely how you would want to see them happen at grandparents' houses, with friends, or during holiday gatherings without the food play that might not be considered good manners in all company. A meal without food play is similar to having a rehearsal for when the individual eats with others without someone present to help facilitate their comfort level. Everyone shows up ready to act like what you want to see happen when you go out with friends, to a restaurant, or over to a family's home for dinner. Remember, our individuals need more practice than most to master a task.

Sensory Spectrum

A person's sensitivity to sensory stimuli is individual along a sliding scale. Many prefer either stimulus that is more or less alerting; however, some have mixed sensory preferences. Drinking room-temperature water is one of the least stimulating experiences to the mouth, while eating a crunchy salt and vinegar potato chip is much more likely to wake up the mouth. To determine where your child's sensitivities fall within this scale, list their accepted or preferred foods, then think about where those foods fall within this spectrum. From this point, brainstorm foods that are similar or have a common texture or ingredient to those on the list. Examples might include spices, herbs, crunchy vegetables, and crunchy snacks. Someone who likes applesauce with cinnamon might be willing to taste yogurt with cinnamon. Finding similarities in foods takes creativity, but it can be a fun, and sometimes challenging, project.

	MOST ALERTING							LEAST ALERTING
SMELL		RANCID	SOUR	SPICY	SAVORY	FRUITY	FRESH	BLAND
SOUNDS		Fizz	Crunch Snap	Grind	Smack	Gulp	Swish	Silent
TASTE			Bitter	Sour	Spicy	Sweet	Savory	Bland
TEMPERATURE			Alternating	Hot	Cold	Cool	Warm	Room Temperature
TEXTURE			Mixed	Crunchy Firm	Ground Soft	Mushy	Puree	Liquid

Figure 5-1
Table by: CEUEspresso and Lemons Nutrition©
Graphic credit: James Lemons, III

Because having a meal involves all our senses, the target stimuli can be unique to eating and mealtime activities, but it doesn't have to be. Improving sensory experiences at mealtime may need to start with having your individual interact in their environment without adding food or drinks to the mix. This process can start with a favorite activity, like conversations, coloring, or puzzles, based on the individual's preferences. Begin by watching to see if they can engage in the activity long enough to complete a meal or snack while simultaneously doing this favorite activity. If there is something in this environment that is a barrier before the food is brought into the picture, evaluate to see if there is a way to change the environment or if there is a strategy to help them deal with the distraction. For example, if there is a noise from a vent or a flickering light, how can this be changed, or what strategies can your individual use to deal with those distractions? Environmental distractions inevitably will happen in places other than at your table. Learning strategies to use in those instances could help them in a classroom or a social gathering. Can they move to a different seat? Can they fidget with an item to help them get through it? Using items generally more accepted in an adult atmosphere has benefits, like fidgeting with prayer beads or wearing sunglasses because the light is hurting their eyes. Sensory work should include being in one spot for a brief time. These skills are necessary for several reasons besides eating, whether standing, sitting in a chair, or sitting on the floor. Kindergarten was challenging for one of my sons and his teacher because he could not sit through circle time, but for eating purposes, it is a skill that is necessary for eating meals in public.

For adults who cannot eat with other people, I start the expansion of their diet by having them eat a meal with someone they trust sitting nearby and then sitting with someone they trust while that person eats. From here, we work on having them eat something simultaneously. Verbal adults may be able to tell you what is causing them discomfort. For non-verbal adults, I watch eye gaze and body language for clues. Once they are comfortable with sitting long enough for a meal or snack, it is time to add food to the environment.

When you look at the meal, you take in the food on the plate, the table, and everything within sight. Perhaps your individual is accustomed to eating peanut butter and grape jelly sandwiches with the crust cut off on a round, blue plate. However, today, they are with someone who only knows they like peanut butter and grape jelly sandwiches. Maybe the crust is still on the bread. Suppose the sandwich is prepared correctly, but presented on a square, yellow plate. In her *SOS Approach to Feeding* course, Kay Toomey encourages families to carry a placemat with them wherever they go so they can consistently use the same placemat for meals. I think this can be an excellent place to start building predictability. However, I encourage future therapy sessions to include other placemats in the regimen to prevent this strategy from becoming like the lost-stuffed-toy nightmare many of us have experienced with our children. Suppose you become dependent on one element to prevent meltdowns. Eventually, something will happen, whether the item is lost or, maybe, damaged to a point the individual insists you "fix it," even though it is beyond restoring. It is also a good idea to work on varying the appearance of the food. Suppose your child will only eat a specific fast-food restaurant's French fries served in their standard container. When the restaurant has a promotion that includes printing the wrapper in a different color, it can cause problems. I have lost count of the families I have known whose children quit eating something due to the change in the wrapper, including my own child. One of my children loved yogurt in tubes. He ate huge amounts of it regularly until they put a cartoon character he didn't like on the label. It has been thirty years, but he still won't eat that food.

When working on changing the appearance of meals, enlist the help of others. I always stick with changing one element at a time. For example, the person sitting the farthest from your child at the table might eat the same meal, but on a different placemat. They might have identical elements on the plate, but have them arranged differently. Or if your individual only accepts regular French fries, the tablemate might have curly fries. I like to ponder possibilities aloud. "Oh look," I might say. "I think I will eat curly fries today and see how those tastes. I wonder if it will taste the same as regular French fries? Yes, it does taste the same; how interesting."

Here is an excellent place to incorporate a story ahead of the meal, discussing how some people like their food to always look orderly, but some people prefer a different look to their food. Your story could conclude that both ways are okay, and everyone has different preferences. Other strategies might include some sensory food play.

Predetermine the boundaries your family wants to place on sensory issue sessions. Are there times when sensory play will not happen, like evening meals, or in the presence of others who may disagree with working through sensory issues? Maybe not during weeks that include overly stressful events or any other limit your family may feel necessary. Determine what sensory play is a priority and concentrate on that priority, then add more priorities when the individual and the family can tolerate it. As we have discussed, overloading a family with therapy is detrimental, and it is easy to overload specific family members who tend to take the heaviest load during these sessions, so it's beneficial to rotate the person working on therapy, if the sensory work at hand requires everyone's participation. Aside from not overloading your therapy partners, you want your individual to eat their newly accepted foods with everyone, not just the one person who always works with them when trying new foods.

Sounds of Foods

One of the commonly overlooked sensory elements associated with food is sound. You might not have given it much thought, but eating creates crunching, squishing, chewing and swallowing sounds, as we saw in Figure 5-1. Most of us know adults who do not have autism and, yet, find the sound of others chewing loudly offensive. Other potentially distracting sounds during meals are typical to the environment. There may be people talking, pans clanging in the kitchen, soft music playing, or arguing at the table. The individuals I work with frequently tell me the sound that distracts them the most is the buzzing of the lights in the room. Adding or omitting sounds to your meals changes the conditions and, therefore, the harmony of the meal. Adjustments to the sounds heard internally from chewing and externally from environmental sounds are made by setting ground rules, using stories, and creating habits that support those rules.

Strategies for dealing with any annoying sounds could be goals incorporated into feeding therapy. Part of that therapy may need to include techniques for chewing quietly. If you prefer instrumental music to set the tone at meals, take incremental steps to include music. Making the intentional presence or lack of music part of mealtime therapy can also help prepare your individual for the countless possibilities of environmental sounds they will need to navigate throughout their lives. The expectation is for our individuals to sit calmly and participate in the social ritual of the meal. Is there a time they will more likely be annoyed or distracted by a sound? In our homes, we may be able to change the environment to fit the needs of our individuals. Even so, they must develop coping methods to integrate into social environments. Coping skills can include asking for reasonable requests, like a volume change, but obtaining those accommodations requires learning the skill of asking politely for what they need.

Texture of Food

The next potential trouble area is texture sensitivity. The feel of food can refer to how it feels to the fingers, lips or tongue, or the sensation the individual receives when the food is pierced or cut with a utensil. There are several ways to increase the foods an individual is willing to touch. I like to start with using utensils or putting food in plastic bags to manipulate without directly touching the food. Please start with the foods your child does accept. If they like Goldfish crackers, crushing those in a plastic bag or between some wax paper with a rolling pin so you can put the crumbs on yogurt, pudding, or applesauce allows them the experience of exploring the texture without feeling threatened. It can also be used instead of sand and glued into an art project. The possibilities are as broad as your imagination. There are great resources to be found in books and magazines, as well as on internet sites such as Pinterest and Instagram.

As already mentioned, exploring all the sensory experiences should be at an individual's pace. Touch is one of the exploration experiences in which we tend to try to push too fast. I said we because I am including myself in wanting to go faster with this one. I find more success, however, if I restrain my desire to go faster and take my time demonstrating and letting the individual repeat the behavior at their comfort level. For example, if I pierce a steamed carrot with a fork, I say something like, "Would you like to try piercing the carrot with a fork?" Even with my adult sons, they will let me know when I push the envelope too far. Along with incorporating their help in the kitchen, I also like using homemade playdough for interaction with food without putting it in their mouth. Rolling pins, apple slicers, and plastic lettuce knives are helpful tools for seeing just how much resistance each item will give when sliced, rolled, and, hopefully, eventually bitten. The goal is to eventually have foods touch the lips, tongue, and teeth.

Imagination play, also, can help accomplish these target goals. In our home, using food as a car, dinosaur, or train would have been the most relevant pretend play to incorporate when working through sensory issues. I had no training when the boys were younger, but I remember playing pretend with food out of sheer desperation. Now, I encourage parents to do it, eventually touching the food to various places on their own body to let their child see how it feels to the adult. Then, if the child doesn't respond negatively, they invite the child to try it. A child who accepts the invitation knowing it is acceptable not to touch their face, cheek, or lips with the food is still making progress. The process of developing trust is the most critical step. They need to know you will not force them to suddenly put an unfamiliar food in their mouth.

Aromas of Foods

The sense of smell is very closely related to taste. When you smell a favorite food, you get a hint of how it will taste in your mouth. Before you're willing to put it into your mouth, you need to be comfortable near the scent. So, how do you acclimate someone to a food's aroma before encouraging a bite? The strategy chosen may depend on whether there is already a negative association with the food. For example, a person may gag merely at the sight of someone picking up cereal from the top of the refrigerator. When the cereal package is opened enough to release the odor, that person might progress to retching. This was a challenge for one of the families I saw for nutrition consultation. As in any progressive therapy, trust must be established before moving forward to work on smell. My goal for an individual with this reaction is for them to be able to stay in the same room while someone eats the cereal.

In this case, I pulled out all my tools. I started with a story discussing how the individual felt about the cereal, how the sibling liked it, and the typical response practiced by the whole family, including discussions on the lack of pressure to eat the food when the sibling took the box from the pantry. In this case, the individual did not need to be in the same room. An excellent place to start is having the sibling stay as far away from the individual as possible. The story reinforced how nobody asked the individual to eat. Still, everyone was proud of him for staying in the adjoining room for a specific number of minutes. These minutes started with one and then moved up with each trial. Working through a strong aversion takes time.

One of my favorite strategies is introducing smells through cooking because the aroma is ambient, not directly exposing the individual to the scent. Let's say you are cooking a food you know your child will not eat. To build trust, ensure they know they don't have to eat it. It may take several tries, but a reasonable goal is to have them sitting at the table without a meltdown while someone else eats foods the individual will not eat. Joining in family or friend gatherings requires sitting at the same table with others without visibly reacting to the food other people eat. Thanksgiving dinner is much more pleasant if little

Johnny isn't gagging while sitting beside Grandma as she eats her favorite pumpkin pie.

Bubbles are a fantastic way to expose someone to a smell. To demonstrate this, I have put coffee extract into bubbles and then given the bubbles to adults, who provide feeding therapy. It is always a hit, and anything water-soluble will dissolve in bubbles. You do need to be prepared to clean up afterward, however. The coffee extract is brown, so testing your bubbles out before doing them at someone's house is a good idea. Many extracts are available for various fruits, but it also works for Grandma's favorite soup if the broth has enough smell to give off an aroma to the bubbles. Presenting smells in a way that causes individuals to reach for the smell instead of turning away, increases the likelihood they will eventually become accustomed enough to eat the associated food.

Tasting Foods

I have saved taste for last because it should be the last piece in the sensory puzzle. Again, every piece of this puzzle needs to be choice versus compliance. Even if you could live forever to always take care of your individual's meal needs, there will be times when they will be with others and have unsupervised access to food. For health reasons, we want our individuals to eat an adequate number of diverse foods, while serving themselves a large enough portion that does not signal, "I'm not going to eat this," before they take the first bite. Variety in the diet ensures they have all the components of nutrition to support good health. Therefore, I encourage portions about the size of a computer mouse for an adult. Since our individuals tend to be perfectionists, I do not encourage precise size or calorie count measurements, as the preoccupation with the precision of caloric intake can lead to eating disorders.

My goal is for the individual to make all the choices without someone hovering over them, trying to influence them. The ability to accomplish tasks without constant supervision applies to all areas of life, including food choices. Our role as caregivers is to encourage good habits using techniques that do not always require our presence. For our sons, the victory is when they can try new foods and eat a balanced meal without us present or when they are sitting at a different table from us in a large group. They are doing well with this goal at this point in their lives. They have learned to explore their curiosity about how different foods taste and to try a little of several different foods at the family or church potluck. They are also confident enough to say things like, "I cannot eat that, it has corn in it," or "I think I will try this food. It looks like something I would like." Seeing others around them enjoying food and making a fuss about the excellent taste increases their chances of trying it exponentially.

While I have some favorite activities for introducing smell, sight, sound, and touch, taste must ultimately be their choice. If you push taste beyond their trust and comfort level, the pushed food rarely becomes something they will enjoy and ask for, much less become their favorite. Tricking someone to eat a food by hiding it in a recipe may "get it down them" occasionally, but doesn't build trust. I prefer to be open. If an individual realizes something they dislike is in the recipe, they most likely will stop eating the food, and if they didn't realize it was in the recipe, they still are unlikely to eat it when you are not hiding it. Frequently, individuals with autism are experts at finding practically invisible specks of ingredients they have no intention of eating, mulling it around in their mouth, swallowing the food they want, then spitting out the speck you thought was well disguised. Almost everyone, with or without autism, can name a food they were pushed to eat, which now they will not eat at all. Forcing your individual to taste something is much more likely to backfire than to be successful. Instead, I prefer to foster curiosity about food and wrap that curiosity in complete trust.

Prepare for Change

Neither the list of foods we can/will eat, nor our health status is static. Sometimes supplies are low in the grocery store, or maybe our financial status changes, and we can no longer afford to buy a favorite brand. Perhaps we develop an intolerance, such as heartburn, celiac disease, etc., to foods we had eaten without problem for years. We cannot count on our favorite prepackaged food recipe nor its packaging never to change. Like all of life, nothing remains the same, and the possibility always exists that our diet will require modification at some point. The ability to embrace a growth mindset when incorporating different foods into our diet is an asset and a vital self-sufficiency skill for our individuals that can provide life-long strong nutritional habits, as well as social and general life competencies.

Chapter Six

Using Stories to Expand Food Selections

When we think of diet and nutrition, we often think about how to restrict our eating habits, but I like to turn that concept around. Nutrition is about how we nourish our bodies. We want the positive effects of eating well, like proper brain development, a strong immune system, the energy to do fun activities, and the satisfaction eating yummy food creates in us. A diverse diet has many benefits, including a healthy gut microbiome that benefits your physical and mental health.

My focus in this chapter is on expanding the list of accepted foods and, therefore, the list of benefits from the nutrition received from food. Balanced diets promote long-term health, but it is hard to achieve when your individual eats only a limited food repertoire, maybe even as few as three food items. If the diet is severely limited, it is impossible to meet protein, vitamins, minerals, and fiber needs. To map out an individual's unique nutritional goals, I always look at where "they are at," as is commonly said in the world of feeding therapy. Here are some questions to ask:

- What do they eat without someone needing to "jump through hoops" to get them to put it in their mouth, chew it, and swallow it without gagging or having some negative reaction?
- What do they ask to eat?
- What is the meal the parents feed them when they need some peace during the meal?
- What sensory elements do the favorite foods have in common? Are they high flavor versus low flavor, and are they crunchy versus smooth and requiring very little chewing?
- Does anyone else who will be present have any sensory

issues with foods, or is anyone else a picky eater?
- Who are the people they will eat with without having a conflict?
- Are these people available to eat with them regularly during feeding therapy sessions?
- Do they stay seated during meals? Is there a trick, or can they sit without extra support if they do?
- Are there any challenges with the meal environment?

I like to start increasing food variety by having the individual eat with those they are comfortable with while eating their favorite foods. Someone should record a video of this meal, so therapists and caregivers can view the video to watch for both skills that should be applauded and areas that need improvement. Using the gathered information, create a plan.

Formulating a Story Plan

I like to write this plan into a story or a series of stories that facilitate working on one challenge at a time. The first question I ask is, "What do you want mealtime to look like?" As parents/caregivers on my caseload talked about how they envisioned mealtime and made those hopes and dreams into a story, I found they modified the story independently when they said something out loud that they realized would be an unrealistic starting point. It also helped them think through their roles at the table while agreeing on ground rules for the meal.

I would return with the story in hand with some clip art added for pictures and a release to take pictures if the family agreed; then, as the story unfolded, we would take photos to be incorporated later. I'd take those images, add them in the appropriate spot, print the story, and return the completed product to the family for later use. Using pictures of the actual people or articles involved in the story, like plates and placemats, seems to make the story more impactful with some kids.

Storytelling is far from being a new strategy to get the point across. There are parables in the Bible for this exact reason. Telling stories allows the listener to see themselves in the story and see that their challenge is being acknowledged. Additionally, stories demonstrate the challenges others in the story may be facing as well, whether that is a mom who is worried her child is not going to eat the only food she can afford or another family member who becomes distressed when the individual has a meltdown at the table.

While the concept of telling stories may feel uncomfortable to you at first, everyone uses the skill on a daily basis, usually without even being aware they are telling a story. From getting out of trouble as children to telling a friend about a recent experience to explaining to the boss why we were late to work, stories knit the fabric of our lives together. My original concept was to use *Social Stories* by Carol Gray (Gray 2010), but I don't do that anymore. Social Stories are a great strategy, and many people working with someone who has autism could probably write some phenomenal stories for individuals and their families; however, I am not very good at Social Stories, as Carol Gray outlines them, so I make up stories that fit my purpose.

After discovering how families want mealtime to look, I include introductions or acknowledgments of all participating in the story. I don't feel it is necessary to introduce every person each time, but I do feel it is important to acknowledge the challenges the individuals present may be experiencing during meals. Those challenges may include the parent's frustration that they have cooked a meal the child does not want to eat. Maybe the parent cannot replace the unwanted food due to finances. It may also include others' frustrations when the child has a meltdown at the table. Be careful to make the story about how the family is going to work through these challenges together and not a scolding about anyone's point of view.

In my stories, I acknowledge other emotions after introducing everyone and their challenges in the meal. This acknowledgment may be that the one trial food is someone else's favorite or one they tried outside of the family and now want everyone else to enjoy so it can be added it to future menus. Someone may have a fear of the food. We acknowledge this and provide alternative methods for trying it. Remember, trying does not mean your individual took a full serving, ate the whole thing, and smiled while they did it. Trying can be putting it on a separate plate and using utensils to investigate the texture by slicing or mashing it. I like to end the story by asking how they might change the recipe in the future.

Stories should include:

- Introduction of those present (a favorite toy can also be an added participant)
- How those individuals fit in the story. Are they feeling challenged by the situation, as well, or maybe you are introducing a food they really like and want others to like as well?
- What is the problem/challenge?
- Write a narrative of how the group will tackle this together.
  - I break out all my sensory strategies here. We use bubbles, food play, pretend meals, and anything I can think of that might work.
- Incorporating the child into the adventure – you can use questions, e.g., Would [enter child's name] like to try it too?
- Appropriate ways to decline if the trial becomes too much

- Appropriate ways to ask for extending the quest if it becomes overwhelming
- Thank everyone for joining in on the fun.

Appropriate Stories

All stories need to be both age and developmentally appropriate. Subjects and discussions in the story need to be at a level your individual can grasp, but also done in a way they do not feel you are treating them as a child much younger than their age. For example, if you are writing a story about cooking skills, you would not want to hand them a knife without adequate safety instruction and demonstration, including how to keep their fingers safe. Writing a story using an apple cutter or lettuce knife instead of a sharp knife to start this journey allows the individual to experience the action of cutting, including the pressure they need to exert, without being exposed to danger. The language used needs to reflect the appropriate maturity level for their age. I recommend wording that models how you would like them to speak as an adult. Speaking to them this way will show respect and your belief that they can handle the barrier that has warranted your attention. Many people with disabilities have voiced their disgust when someone presents them with information written for children, complete with childish pictures. My preference for materials and stories used to address obstacles our individuals face is always to create those materials specifically for them. I realize there is not always time to create something unique to their needs, but I would rather see an oral story told that is age-appropriate and has no printed aids, than to use materials that are not age or developmentally appropriate.

Too Old for Stories?

I work with adults with autism who have been willing to write their own stories about food challenges. Our boys are adults, advanced in their willingness to be adventurous while trying novel foods, and they have outgrown stories. So, we have a casual conversation about the food, how it smells, how to check out its texture, and acceptable ways to decline future bites. If it is a food I do not expect to be eaten as a full serving, or is not usually eaten as a full serving, like pickles, I serve it as an addition to the meal instead of a replacement for one of their preferred foods, but we do not make another meal because the boys did not like what I served. The benefit to having done this for quite a long time at this point is we usually have a good idea of how far we can push these trials and still ensure everyone has enough food.

Next Steps

Future steps include writing follow-up stories – or in my family's case, having a conversation – about trying the food in another form. While your child may love hamburgers from fast food restaurant A, they may have never tried hamburgers from fast food restaurant B or from your favorite sit-down restaurant that happens to have a child's menu. Trying foods in different forms can be trying burgers from those other places or trying cheeseburgers instead of hamburgers. We pick a food to try, (well, to be honest, most of the time I pick it. Let's just say taking a vote usually results in foods that do not increase variety a lot.)

Anyway, we pick a food that the boys do not eat and maybe have never tried. We use different cooking methods like baked, air-fried, or broiled. I usually do not fry in oil, but that is largely due to not wanting to deal with the mess or the nutritional impact of fried foods. I also want to keep techniques that the boys can employ on the nights they cook for the family, and I have not tackled fried foods with them. One of our trials was pickles. We did the obvious first; we had slices of pickles straight out of the jar. Next, we made hot dogs and added pickle relish. I then used relish in a recipe and finally made fried pickles and had ranch dressing available. In this case, the ranch dressing was not officially part of the trial as it was a new food, also. Overall, the trial was a complete bust as far as adding new foods, but if we take a step back and look at how far we have come even to be able to add something like pickles, which have a stronger flavor than either of the boys usually like and they willingly participated, then I move this to the success column.

Stories might include how to communicate gratitude to others for the offer of food while declining to eat it. Yet another may include incorporating your individual in the kitchen chores to give them more control over food preparation and teach them new kitchen skills. Some stories may have nothing to do with a particular food, but rather how to handle food outside the home, whether they like that food or not. A priority might be using stories to describe eating appropriate amounts of food at a family gathering, so your individual knows the difference between putting so small an amount of food on their plate that it insults the cook versus taking a huge portion that would make it impossible for others in attendance to have a chance to enjoy it. Hopefully, you can find a way to use stories to bring peace and joy to your meals.

Contingency Plans

Everyone has emergencies and spur-of-the-moment changes in their life. We take CPR and First Aid classes with the hope of never needing to use the knowledge, but it's important to learn the steps so we can better handle an emergency, if it arises. I encourage you to write stories that prepare your children for situations that will disrupt their predictable routine. When those occasions happen, your child will likely need to be with someone other than you for a period. It will make the emergency much easier to deal with if you are not also dealing with the aftermath of a meltdown and possibly a child who did not eat anything because the food they were offered was wrong for them. Think through what behaviors or habits you are encouraging or protecting to keep some much-needed peace in your daily lives. Some examples from our lives include:

- One of our boys always sitting on the left of everyone because he is left-handed, whether it is in the car, at the table, or in a group.
- Allowing certain toys, like a truck in our case, to be kept in a specific place because that is where they felt it belonged
- Meals occurring at a specific time
- Eating French fries, but putting the longest off to the side and eating that longest one last
- Eating Smarties candy by counting the number of candies

after each bite

- Sleeping with specific toys
- Eating the chocolate off the peanut M&Ms
- Eating only chicken and flavored gelatin when dining out
- Insisting on eating at a restaurant to get a specific toy
- Having conversations between their imaginary dinosaurs (each hand was a dinosaur) no matter what was going on around them
- Foods were not allowed to be touching.

You can probably think of times when all of these habits would have been a challenge that needed to be resolved, but Richard's teacher tells the story about his ever-present dinosaurs being a severe disruption to learning. She struggled for a solution until she happened on the idea of having him put the dinosaurs inside his desk during instruction. He resisted some, but she persevered and eventually, the dinosaurs learned to come out only during the times she had designated as being okay. For Jason, the big challenge was insisting on sitting on the left. One day he needed to ride somewhere with a friend because of a family emergency. There were tears and a meltdown due to the seating not fitting his usual pattern. The problem was rooted in the fact others did not understand the logic in his devotion, plus his need for this accommodation was counterproductive to the situation. These specific challenges are some we have looked back on and wished we had known about the tool of writing stories. All of us, the boys included, feel a story might have helped us work through these challenges more quickly.

While situations will eventually happen that throw your child right out of their comfort zone, there is also the possibility of natural disasters, sudden family emergencies like a grandparent having a health event, or personal emergencies like a fire in the house. Consider your own situation and decide what events you might want to discuss. Two possibilities are natural disasters depending on where you live and possible family emergencies based on any current health issues of those you love.

My First Food Story

The following represents the first story I wrote with a family. I have changed names and several conditions for privacy reasons. I knew time was short to help this family. They had just received an autism diagnosis for their child, and he was not eating much of anything. I was a brand-new dietitian, excited to take on the challenge and armed with the knowledge I had gained as a parent of two boys with autism. I had seen this family a few times and knew a few things about the challenges of feeding their son, who we will call Daniel. He had gone through a period of eating only round foods, he loved to watch the trash truck, and he loved the movie, *Toy Story*. For my part, I had my own challenges. The experienced occupational therapist I had anticipated learning the ropes from had suddenly retired. In her place was a brand-new graduate with no experience beyond her education and very little knowledge of autism. In an effort to make a difference for this child before he aged out of our program in three short months, I pitched the idea of trying Carol Gray's Social Story method. I had learned about this technique, but had never actually written a

Story. The one I wrote fell incredibly short of qualifying for meeting the specified requirements, but my concept was the same. I wrote a straightforward story narrating the therapy session with personal touches added that would allow everyone to relax and act out the story without having a professional dictate what they needed to do.

The brand-new OT and I came armed with our story, pretzel sticks, and peanut butter dip. My colleagues thought I had lost my marbles but were willing to humor me for the moment. In any case, snacks and Daniel's favorite toys would be involved.

I began the story by saying, "Daniel's friend, Miss Cyndi, has come to play with him today. She brought snacks for Daniel and her to eat. First, Miss Cyndi has fruit roll-ups to try. She is going to put one end of the fruit roll-up in her mouth and one end in Daniel's mouth, then they'll eat towards each other."

As Daniel and Cyndi acted out the story, I could see he was firmly hooked, so I continued it. "Miss Sharon brought some yummy dip with peanut butter, cool whip, and cinnamon." Pointing to Daniel's favorite toy, I said, "Maybe Woody would like to try some." Daniel stuck Woody's hand in the dip with one prompt and immediately sucked the dip off Woody's hand.

"Now," I said, "maybe Buzz would like to try some dip." Daniel plunged Buzz's hand into the dip, pulled it out and sucked the goo off Buzz's hand.

Next came the big test. Would Daniel like to try the dip? Cyndi and I turned our attention to reaching for a pretzel stick and a baby wipe so Daniel, who didn't like getting his hands dirty, could taste the dip comfortably, and his hands could be cleaned the moment anything accidentally got on them. When we turned back to Daniel, he had plunged his hand to the bottom of the bowl, proudly lifting it out, and licked it off his fingers. Success! The parents informed me he would not eat anything without that dip for weeks.

While this was the first story I used as a professional, it definitely was not the last. I quickly discovered my idea of getting Daniel to try new foods was a little overwhelming to the parent's own sensory issues. From then on, I asked if others had sensory issues before I started the story.

As you think about stories, what foods can you link to your individual's accepted foods? The book *Food Chaining: The Proven 6-Step Plan to Stop Picky Eating, Solve Feeding Problems, and Expand Your Child's Diet* (Fraker, et al. 2007) details many ways to link those foods. I especially like linking textures and flavors, but I also like incorporating food play outside meals. I encourage you to think about how to expand the foods your individual will eat into other food groups. Often, I see this method used only for linking one carbohydrate to another and then yet another. Remember, we are working towards wellness, so all food groups are needed.

As you successfully add more menu items without undue stress, remove any duplicates. For example, replace those ever-present chicken nuggets with other proteins when new foods are added successfully. The goal is to have a meal plan that includes as much variety as possible, using as many different textures and colors as possible.

That said, while I have seen recommendations to completely stop offering the "go-to" food items, the individual will always ask to eat them. I don't encourage a sudden, total removal of any food unless it is for a medical reason. A complete removal will add too much stress. Dietary changes need to be gradual in anyone's life, much less in a family with many other challenges. Also, remember that being transparent about new foods and textures is crucial while building confidence. Families who make it a habit to reveal how foods are different from those already accepted and give permission not to eat what the child doesn't like increase the possibility of trying new foods. Using a story is a great, non-threatening way to talk with your individual about untried foods.

Like everything else with autism, stories need to be individualized. But is it always necessary for the stories to be presented in the exact same format? Do they always need to be written out and printed with appropriate thoughtful pictures to effectively work through challenges? I don't know about anyone else, but the thought that I needed to put that much work into every single intervention was a huge barrier to me when incorporating stories into our daily life. Part of the goal of using stories is keeping the process pleasant but productive. With a bit of practice, you may be able to do this without writing the story out. I promise you the storytellers I knew growing up never wrote a story down, but today we have tools of convenience the old-time storytellers did not. Using video recordings may be a much easier way to add stories into your routines, and today's technology makes it easy to make follow-up videos of your efforts. In fact, videos are useful whether the story is written or not. You can always look back and watch everyone's body language to see where a strategy really took off or where it broke down.

Whether you create simple stories with words alone, or you make them more elaborate with photos and videos, my advice to you is to give it a try. The results can prove revolutionary in small ways that make huge differences to you, your family and your individual. Whatever you do, relax, look forward with optimism to solving some of your struggles, laugh, and have fun.

Chapter Seven

Special Diets

My initial response to realizing Richard, my oldest, would need some intervention was to try a dietary approach before putting my four-year-old on medications. The doctor's office I called for assistance told me they did not discuss dietary solutions. I didn't even give them my name and hung up. We went on for a while trying to implement our own changes before someone encouraged me to at least hear what the doctors had to say. They offered neither a dietary approach nor medication, but they steered me towards educational strategies while encouraging a visit to the allergist. During this first visit was when they also told me he would probably never hold a pencil. I'm proud to say today he has an associate degree in graphic arts and a bachelor's degree in media arts and animation. In fact, he is the artist for all the graphic artwork in this book, including the cover, further emphasizing the point I frequently make: We need to quit practicing crystal-ball medicine because we do not have one.

Allergies

We took the physicians' advice and did go to the allergist, but didn't hold any hope that treating allergies would "fix" our son. The allergist agreed; however, she still wanted to do the testing, based on two physical symptoms. Richard had the worst "allergic shiners" she had seen in a long time, and she noticed he quickly gave the "allergic salute." For those not familiar with these phrases, I'll give a little context: Allergic shiners are dark circles under the eyes that indicate sinus pressure. I always thought it was because he did not get enough sleep, which was also true. If he could wiggle a toe, he could stay awake. The "allergic salute" is when an individual wipes their nose with the palm of the hand moving straight up past the forehead. The doctor laughed and said, "Salute!" as he did it. Toddlers frequently learn to wipe their noses in this manner if their nose runs quite a lot.

The allergen scratch test on Richard's back resulted in immediate and intense reactions. He began to shake and cry, and I cried with him and held him. Almost everything they tested was a four-quadruple-plus on a scale of one to four. Three foods were positive on his test: corn, soy, and peanuts. If I had known then what I know now about food allergies, I would have been more scared, but at that point, I did not know anything about them. The internet was not around yet, and books on the topic were few and far between. This event also happened a decade before I returned to school to become a dietitian.

Second Visit

When the allergist told me to remove the allergens and then add them back into the diet one at a time, I did it without question. We also started Richard on shots and daily antihistamines. He was a changed child. Before treating his allergies, he was in constant motion. He would swing his hands and make noises with his mouth while he paced over and over up and down the hall, a stimming behavior not unusual for autism. He could not concentrate enough to play with toys that would typically be used to keep a child quiet. As soon as we started treating his allergies with antihistamines, he stopped stimming completely and could suddenly play with some of those quiet toys to occupy himself. Frankly, I did not believe what I saw. I went to each person who spent significant periods with Richard and asked what they thought. We all agreed he was a different child. I did not expect the allergist to believe me when I returned, so I asked each person to write a letter. Gathering all the letters, I returned to the follow-up appointment with the child and the letters in hand. Without saying anything, I handed the letters to the doctor, who read each one. When She handed them back to me, she said, "You did not expect me to believe you." She was correct; I did not.

We discussed how the shots were going, his nightly antihistamine, and the foods. As instructed, I removed soy, corn, and peanuts. As I added each back into his meals, I saw his ability to concentrate and have good impulse control change only with the addition of corn. Soy and peanuts seemed not to affect his behavior or his health.

The total lack of stimming and improved concentration did not last permanently. Some of his symptoms returned as soon as we turned on the heater. He was walking down the hall like any other typical child when the heater turned on, but by the time he reached the other end of the hall, he was flapping his hands and making noise again. It never returned to the previous intensity, but it did return. This gave us some significant clues into his behavior from that point forward. We knew if the wind was blowing or the pollen count was high, he would struggle with self-control on those days. This was also true when he ate anything with corn. As an adult he can now report to us that this is due to both the overstimulation from the sound of the wind and the overwhelming effects of the allergens in the air.

Testing the Corn Theory

Just to be certain, we tried the corn theory several times. I called the Autism Research Institute where Bernard Rimland, the founder, answered the phone himself on the second ring. He advised me not to tell anyone when I made changes to Richard's diet, except those who specifically needed to know. So, I followed his advice, telling none but those in the need-to-know circle. As for those outside that circle, even though these adults were not told about the diet changes, they could always identify any time I allowed him to have some corn. Every single grandparent, church worker, or school personnel recognized something was different; they didn't know what, but his behavior was so different they would comment on it. As a grown-up, Richard still has reactions to corn. Today, it goes something like this: "Richard, you seem distracted. What did you eat this morning?" When he brings me the label, I show him the corn product listed. There have been a few times when Richard has decided that as an adult, he no longer needs to pay attention to that "allergy stuff." This has resulted in some cases of esophagitis which we discovered when he had eaten corn and, then, later when he tried to swallow other food, it became stuck on the way down requiring intervention. During one emergency room visit they retrieved the piece of food, and during another they administered medication to relax his esophagus sufficiently for the food to pass. Until these frightening experiences happened, we had not realized just how dangerous his corn allergy was.

Autism Diet

When Richard was young, like many families, we wanted to do a less invasive intervention that would not require our oldest child to be on drugs from a young age. We naively expected to find that there was a particular diet that worked to mitigate the issues our child was having. In other words, we felt we must be feeding him wrong, in general, or he wouldn't be having these challenges. The last problem we expected to find was that he had food allergies. I have had opportunities during my career to have brief conversations with food allergy researchers, and they all are adamant that food allergies do not cause autism. I agree, but they and I have all been willing to concede that a child dealing with food allergies, intolerances, or seasonal allergies will have less success compensating for any autism traits they are trying to control, just like you and I have more difficultly dealing with our daily stresses when we have a headache.

Sometimes people ask what I think of the autism diet. My response is always, "Which autism diet?" There is a long list of foods that professionals often recommend restricting from the diets of all children with autism. Personally, I have never been a fan of the "shotgun approach," in which parents base restrictions on a long list of potential offenders or take a single theory on food. Basically, they are shooting the problem with every possible solution all at once. The issue with this approach is if you try a multitude of strategies all at once and the problem improves, you do not know which strategy worked.

Individuals with autism are frequently picky or problem eaters who already severely limit their food. By removing a predetermined list of foods that might or might not impact their behavior, we are also removing potential sources of nutrition their other preferred foods may not provide. Healthful diets include calories, protein, carbohydrates, fiber, vitamins, and minerals for achieving appropriate growth to support physical and mental health, as well as brain development. A diet that does not hit all these marks is inadequate and must be improved. However, no diet is perfect, nor should we ever push for perfection when feeding a child. Stressing perfection in a diet encourages eating disorders.

Any problems with particular foods or food components like gluten, casein, soy, sugar, eggs, particular oils, or many other ingredients should be evaluated by your child's medical team. This team should include a dietitian to evaluate for any potential nutritional deficiencies. I prefer to determine if, and when, foods need to be eliminated by evaluating a person's reactions to those foods and whether there is a documented adverse reaction resulting from medical testing which indicates the food should be removed. Like every other intervention in autism, all interventions should be individualized. In Richard's case, if allergy testing had not been recommended, and his restrictions called for a casein-free, gluten-free diet, which is frequently recommended for autism, I would have typically replaced the gluten with corn, the exact opposite of what he actually needed.

Elimination of foods does not ensure a healthy diet; it only makes it more difficult to balance the diet. While gluten may be a food source that causes challenges for some, it is important to remember when removing this nutrient that many sources of gluten-containing foods are fortified with important vitamins and minerals. If gluten is removed from a diet, then the breads and cereals that provide fortified vitamins and minerals must be obtained from another source. The best strategy for including all the vitamins and minerals needed by growing children is to eat a diverse group of foods, which is very difficult with finicky eaters since many eat as few as three foods. Eating a balanced diet while adhering to a person's food restrictions can be done, but it is often a huge amount of work. Moreover, restricting certain foods may sound like an easy fix for someone's challenges, but it is not.

When the gluten-free, casein-free diet became popular for autism, I talked to my boys about the possibility of this diet since they were old enough to acquire their own food when they were at school. If we were going to try it, I needed them to buy into the concept. They did not! The only question they asked was, "Can I still eat pizza?" We were basically done with that discussion.

Again, food restrictions should be addressed with the medical team, which may include allergists, gastroenterologists, dietitians, or others. In addition, if your child is old enough to get food from other places like school parties or other social gatherings, they need to buy into the concept to make it work. If you do try a special diet, I always encourage regular evaluations of how beneficial it is to continue. How often you evaluate that is up to you and your family. Reasons to discontinue might include meeting the required diet costs more than the budget can support, having an accidental food exposure that did not result in the negative effects you had expected, or there is frequent "cheating." Reasons to continue would include: accurately being able to identify when an accidental exposure has taken place, an improvement in symptoms previously present when the food had been included in the diet, and an expected adverse physical reaction to the eliminated food when accidental exposure happens.

A Word about Supplements

Along with diets, I am frequently asked which supplements I recommend. The answer is I do not recommend any. The perception is that supplements are natural, therefore, they are safe. The reality is that supplements can and do have side effects. These side effects are not listed on the bottles, because supplements are not federally regulated and there is no law requiring the side effects be listed. Any time someone takes a supplement they should research possible side effects and discuss them with the individual's medical team to avoid medication reactions with the supplements.

Isolation

Our social lives revolve around food and drinks, so it follows that restricting foods can cause many problems. One of the challenges families who have children with special needs often eventually face is isolation, especially if there is a behavioral factor like autism to their diagnosis. Food restrictions can intensify this. Children with food challenges frequently are not invited to parties or group activities with their peers. More than one person has said to me, "Sharon, you understand why we can't invite Richard. It is just too hard for everyone to worry about his food allergy." In fact, no, I do not understand, but I do comprehend that others feel this way. Isolation does not apply only to children's activities, though. Family gatherings and those with the parents' social groups can also be impacted for the same reason. The lack of inclusion by these social groups is tough for families. Some families report that dealing with food restrictions causes as much of a challenge as having a family member with cancer.

Suppose you are a friend or family member who wants to

change this for another. Good for you! I applaud you. So how do you accomplish this? I'm glad you asked. Family and friends can help set up a safe space for their loved ones who need special diets. The most critical part of this process is setting boundaries on comments and judgment towards either the person who needs the food restrictions or others in their family. I am always glad to help educate someone on Richard's food allergy. Still, I have very little tolerance for anyone judging him or me in a setting that should be a safe emotional haven for our family. I don't waste my time arguing with someone who doesn't believe he needs those accommodations, but I can quickly set a boundary by telling others the subject is not up for discussion. I do not feel the need to defend my decisions as a parent to everyone who disagrees. While everyone should make their own decisions concerning those in their care, it is not necessary to defend those decisions with everyone.

As a host, making sure some of the food at your gathering meets the needs of a family who has a child with food restrictions is a great strategy to make them feel welcome. Even better, see to it that the "special" food is something delicious that everyone is likely to eat, so the individual can see others enjoying their same food. Ensure seating arrangements include people who understand the individual's needs and can redirect conversation away from their restricted diet. Choosing someone outside the immediate family for this position will not only help the individual diversify both their diet and their social network, it allows the family a much-needed respite from always being "on duty" so they can enjoy socializing, as well.

Spending Time with Friends

In working towards well-adjusted social lives that promote wellness and connectedness, the one element I cannot provide for my children is time spent with others who enjoy and seek out their company. Social time outside our immediate family needs to be externally initiated. While this does not happen perfectly in our world, it probably does not happen perfectly in anyone else's world, either. We have been fortunate enough to have some in our lives who have taken on this role, and just like everyone else's social circle, those who are part of that circle come and go. This change is also a typical part of life. Navigating all these changes in life and relationships are essential to the boys' future autonomy. Being connected to others and really feeling that connection in life has many benefits not only to physical wellness, but emotional and mental wellness as well.

Chapter Eight

You Don't Have to Be Perfect

When our house was on the market with our new home soon to be move-in ready, we needed to keep it "house-hunter ready" and be able to vacate with very little notice for showings while continuing to live in it and take care of our daily needs, like eating and cooking. Jason was always the first home and had come to love cooking and doing things for the family, so I bought a couple of those "meal-in-a-bag" dinners for him to cook as soon as he got home.

I fully admit I should have vetted the ingredients a little better, but as any busy parent can attest, sometimes small details are missed, and some of these one-bag menu options I bought definitely fell into the cracks. One day, I notified Jason that he needed to prepare dinner when he got home, and he gladly complied. After a long day at work, I came rushing in the door to dish up the food he had proudly prepared for everyone and stopped short when I realized it had broccoli. And not just a little broccoli, either. Broccoli was one of the major ingredients, and there were good-sized pieces! This was a lapse in my usual diligence to ensure everything we ate would be acceptable to the whole family, since broccoli was not anyone's favorite. More accurately, it was on most everyone's list of "I'll have something else, *please*." Totally convinced that very little of it would be eaten, I scooped portions for everyone into bowls. As I took my bowl and sat at the table, I realized Jason had eaten every bite. Astonished, I looked at him and said, "Jason, you ate all the broccoli! Did you like it?" He responded, "No, but Coach told me broccoli was good for me, so I ate it."

This experience is a great illustration of how things can work out, even when we are not perfect in carrying out our parental duties. Having teachers and other professionals who come alongside you to encourage and mentor your child helps fill in the gaps and gives your individual a wider circle. Coach was someone Jason liked, and the feeling was mutual. He eventually presented Jason with his robe when he graduated from high school. Jason's close bond with Coach translated into an easy willingness to try a food that might never have been tried without considerable work on our part.

I always felt that everything I did as a parent needed to be perfect. Of course, that is unrealistic, but I think most parents of special needs children feel pressured to achieve the same perfection. For pity's sake, every misstep in our children's behavior is under the microscope to a point I did not even know was possible before autism entered our lives! Our children are evaluated for what happened before the behavior (including what might have happened at home beforehand), the moment of the behavior, the sensory environment they were in, and then "the behavior." By the time that process was completed for every infraction, I felt more than inadequate. If you are a parent, please give yourself a break. If you are a professional, strive to help families and the individuals you work with to accept the idea that it is okay not to be perfect.

Change the Narrative!

Since neither we, our children, nor anyone else will ever reach that heightened state, let's discuss dealing with imperfections. Humans mourn their mistakes and shortcomings, but I encourage you to count your successes, instead. I always craved any positive word indicating the boys were progressing. I doubt I am unique among parents of individuals with autism or any other parent group. If you allow yourselves to concentrate only on what is not going "right," you are setting yourself up for depression, anxiety, and frustration. I'm not saying to view your world through rose-colored glasses, but don't dwell on the problems. Remember the statistic in the first chapter that shows those with autism have a higher incidence of mental health issues? So do their parents. We want to model for our children practices that promote our own good mental health, then discuss the reasons and processes with them, teaching them good self-care habits. While the individual is without question the most important person on the team, their parents and caregivers are their most important support. They are the gatekeepers to the individual and their commitments, including how much time they devote to educational work versus social and life skills. That said, here's a reminder to the professionals who work with us to benefit our individuals: it is extremely helpful and encouraging when we hear from you that other parents are not perfect, either, and that we are doing a great job.

Therapy-Free Meals

As you read this book, you will notice I say more than once that every meal should not be therapy. There are multiple reasons for this, but primarily, it's not realistic. If mealtime is always therapy-time, our individuals will not learn how to handle themselves when no one facilitates their actions. Of course, these non-therapy meals won't have perfect interactions, but neither will they if you try to make each meal a therapy session. There will be times when you need to adjust to changing circumstances, but the way to know what your individual has genuinely learned is to allow them to do the skill without prompting. They will need to be able to continue independently with the abilities they have learned when eating in public situations, among friends, and in family gatherings, to name a few.

Therapy-free meals also allow you to make notes about what needs to happen next, which skills they need to learn next on their path to independence and, maybe, even to being adventurous in the kitchen. What social skills need to be practiced and which were done well and should be praised to help those competencies grow? Most importantly, it demonstrates to your individual that meals do not have to be, nor should they be, rigid. Meals can be predictable and comfortable, a time of enjoyment and relaxation. This will take time and devotion to accomplish, but it can be done.

Changing Circumstances

Therapy meals, specific routines, and visual cues prepare your individual for situations utilizing practiced habits that provide the predictability those with autism crave. However, nothing stays the same forever, but even a change in labeling can throw off meals when individuals expect to see their preferred food in the same package as always. Consider the incident I mentioned earlier in the book where I talked about the time a food company changed the look of Jason's favorite yogurt package. It took us a while to find a suitable replacement for the brand. The same phenomenon can happen for many reasons including maybe the plate your individual eats on is different now, the company changed their recipe, and their food has a different texture and taste or, perhaps, the company that makes your individual's favorite food went out of business. How do you feel when one of your favorite foods disappear because the company stopped making it or your favorite restaurant took it off the menu? Even adults sometimes struggle with their favorite products changing. In my family, we prevent these challenges from becoming an issue by working on how to handle regular changes. While we allow ourselves to relax and enjoy routines and predictability, we also include some changes as part of the routine. Sometimes that even means something as simple as removing the offending item from our selections.

Building in Some Unpredictability

As the adage says the only constant is change. Intentionally sprinkling change into your routines can help your individual better deal with the big changes that may come. We have Taco Tuesday at our house, a weekly ritual initiated by Jason. I'm not sure whether he saw Taco Tuesday advertised at a restaurant or heard someone he liked talking about it, but for whatever reason, he decided he wanted to have tacos every Tuesday. Sometimes we have tacos with corn or flour tortillas, accompanied by corn chips and queso dip. At other times, we make taco rings using taco meat and cheese wrapped in canned crescent roll dough. Tuesday is the one day a week I do not insist everyone eat a non-carbohydrate vegetable. I may have a salad with taco meat to accommodate my nutrition needs or eat what everyone else eats, but everyone is given flexibility on Tuesday. I use Taco Tuesday to demonstrate that everything does not have to be the same for each meal. Moreover, everything does not have to be the same for each person, at any of our meals. While I want to see my sons add those non-carbohydrate vegetables to meals, it does not have to happen every time we eat. When we went on vacation, we could eat something different on Tuesday without meltdowns or stress, and while we did eat tacos on vacation, it did not happen on a Tuesday.

Health Issues

Like everyone else, sometimes during physician visits we are told we have to adjust what we eat. Skinny does not mean healthy, nor does it mean all your labs will be good. Jason is over six feet and is now up to about 130 pounds. At one point, he wore 27 x 36 pants. My husband wore 29 x 36 pants and weighed 126 pounds when we got married. Jason's build has much more to do with genetics than limiting calories. He can outeat all of us. He also rides his bicycle several miles a day, which helps keep him thin. In spite of these positive factors, he has begun to have higher cholesterol readings. Altering food choices because of labs is reasonably new to Jason.

On the other hand, Richard has always needed some restrictions in his diet because of his food allergies. As time goes on, and the most recent labs indicate some changes in diet are needed, we adjust. Altering their diet according to what is happening with your individual's health is a critical skill. As I have previously discussed, there is a greater likelihood of several diseases, including heart disease and diabetes, in people with autism. The focus on nutrition needs to be about nourishing our bodies to promote good health and provide energy to do the body's work, so adjusting what we eat for health reasons is a part of life. In fact, this is the very reason we work on expanding food choices. If the work to introduce food variety is done before a change is mandated by medical reasons, then making those alterations when the lab work comes back with issues is much easier on everyone. When faced with a change of diet due to health reasons, many people tell me, "If it tastes good, I can't have it." While it's generally possible to work through the list of preferred foods to help someone come to peace with diet changes, it is much easier if they have a longer list of food preferences to start with, as opposed to a short list.

Methods for Dealing with an Unfamiliar Food

Since change is inevitable, whether circumstantially or mandated by medical professionals, the most effective strategy I have found for coping with change is to work through some methods for handling those alterations when they occur. For this we try to develop systems ahead of time. For dealing with the unexpectedness when a food that is new to the individual is on the menu, our process looks like this:

1. Acknowledge you are unfamiliar with the food.
2. Ask questions about the food. What is in it? Is it spicy? Which spices or herbs are in it? Is it chewy, crunchy, or soft? (Each person may have specific questions they want answered according to preferences.)

Note: If someone is unwilling to answer these questions, it is acceptable to stop here and say, "I don't eat food that I know nothing about." Taking this stance may mean your child pulls out foods they keep handy if there is nothing else they like available or, perhaps, does not eat at all. Some people will not like this stance; that's okay. The goal is to have a balanced, healthy diet while maintaining a good relationship with food. I see the ability to tell someone no as setting boundaries.

3. After acquiring information about the food, individuals need to determine if they will try it. They should feel free to obtain a full-sized portion if there are enough features about the food they like. If they are uncertain they will like it, but have reached the point where they are comfortable trying most everything, they may want to say "I want to try a smaller portion, first," and try a bite or two. Taking one bite and saying, "No, I don't like that," should not be a problem in a supported situation.

Crisis

One of my favorite lines from the character Bones in Star Trek is, "The more you overthink the plumbing, the easier it is to stop up the drain." While setting up routines and keeping life as predictable as possible can help things rock along more smoothly, it does not always work. Everyone encounters a crisis at some point. A crisis can be huge, consisting of something like a natural phenomenon, such as a tornado. Some crises are mundane and a matter of personal perspective, such as forgetting to buy one of the ingredients you need for a meal. In either case, your routine for the day includes something unexpected and your planned activity may be affected. Having contingency plans, which was covered in Chapter 7, can make the crisis much less of an ordeal. Stories are always a good place to start this process. Sit down and write out a list of obstacles that could derail the calm of your day, and work on stories that will help you get through those times. You might start with something you know will likely happen.

I always find it interesting when challenges that come to

everyone's life, like a family illness or even car trouble, happen to us, and then someone comments on our family experiencing more than our share of bad luck. While I might wish that having two individuals in our home who happen to have autism would exempt us from experiencing the same challenges everyone has, it does not, but we have become pretty adept at handling the unexpected. Our whole family learned to be prepared for the unexpected from participating in Scouts. The boys participated in a lot of practice scenarios, while James and I were leaders of the activities. At this point, when the unexpected comes, everyone gets an assignment, and we all know the others are counting on us to do our parts to get through whatever crisis has happened. A couple of years ago, James' mother was having a crisis on Richard's birthday, and we were expecting company to share some cake with us. While James rushed to handle his mother's crisis, I needed to pick up something for that night, and we still needed to go get a cake. Jason was at home cooking the hamburger patties, so I took Richard and sent him in to go pick his own birthday cake. Taking our cue from standup comedian

Jeff Foxworthy's "you might be a redneck if" spiel, we said, "You might be an adult when mom sends you in with the debit card to buy your own cake on your birthday." What defines us is not the number of challenges we face, but how we face our challenges.

Chapter Nine

Medical Wellness

You might remember my earlier story about our son Jason's dental misadventures, but let's return to the topic for a moment. When we initially realized he had a dental problem, we dutifully took him to the dentist where we were told to our horror that *every single tooth in his mouth had decayed*. The least number of cavities in any tooth was three, but most teeth were seventy-five to ninety-percent eroded. Our insurance would not pay for this work to be done in the hospital, so our dentist placed a call to the insurance company in which he lost his temper and told them that if he did this in the office, the insurance company would need to pay for psychiatric treatment for Jason, his mother, and him! They did not budge. He eventually led us to apply for a grant program to have the work completed in the hospital.

What followed that conversation was not the finest hour for anyone involved, so I'll spare you the details. Still, it did teach us a valuable lesson—wellness care, including dental, needed to be a priority. The top priority was preparing the boys to understand and accept the help that was being provided by their medical teams. Over thirty years later, we still ensure everything is explained, and that both the provider and the boys are comfortable before any treatment starts.

As the boys have reached adulthood, it has been essential they handle as much of their wellness as possible. Of course, it is on our minds that one day we will not be able to help with this process, but there have been other priorities, too. The most humanly universal of the reasons is time constraints. Besides our work responsibilities and personal commitments, life has happened around here. My husband and I both have careers. We, also, spent quite a few years prioritizing the care of our elderly parents. Forming strong relationships with the different medical teams, each other, and the boys has been key to making sure our sons' health needs are met, even during our most busy personal seasons.

For all medical appointments dealing with a newly arisen medical issue, one of us will take off from work to be there as a second set of ears. Of course, this is always a good idea for any family; the practice is not unique to autism. One of our current priorities is teaching our sons how to identify and ask for assistance from a trusted friend or family member who can fill this role if we are unable to do it or are unavailable at the moment. Past the first visit, we let the boys handle as many of the appointments as they can on their own. We are listed on all their HIPPA forms. The providers know in advance of their visits that they will be coming alone, but we are available by phone. We also have set up a relationship where the provider will either call us while the boys are there or contact us afterward to let us know if there is an issue that needs to be discussed. We prefer, however, to have the boys explain the issue as they understand it, then we can contact the provider if we need clarification.

Whether we have just been lucky to find providers that naturally work well with this system or those who are willing to put in the extra effort to make our strategy successful does not matter, but we have those relationships in place. I encourage writing letters of introduction that identify some of the challenges your individual may face in cooperating with their medical team and giving these to all new providers ahead of the appointment time. See the sample letter in the appendix.

Keeping Up with Scheduled Appointments

One of the most daunting challenges for maintaining wellness seems to be keeping up with how often appointments and testing should be repeated. Daily I talk to people who have let these tasks slip by to the point they feel embarrassed enough they don't want to "face the music" and talk to their healthcare provider about it, or they have become afraid of the results, so they just don't want to do it. Regardless we all need to have strategies for keeping up with these tasks. If people exist who never let a routine blood test or checkup slip by without getting it done, I am not counted among them. The only way I can keep up with all these tasks or teach anyone else to do so is to make a schedule. Electronic calendars can be very helpful but are not without flaws. If an appointment drops out of my calendar, it may be quite a while before I remember to return to it. In the following pages, I have included samples of organizational charts that I use with my family. The plain truth is that none of us live forever. The more we can do to prepare our individuals for successful and healthy independence, the better for them and for our own peace of mind. I have included a variety of basic charts I use with my family. These are here for reference only, but remember, everyone's health is individual, and you will need to create your own versions of these, based on the advice of your medical team. You might have more providers, or those on your list might have a different frequency for recommended screenings. While many people with diabetes require a blood test every three months, someone without any identified health conditions may need only one test annually. The most important thing to remember is that achieving optimum wellness for yourself and your family is not a matter of accident, but of intent. When there are so many other pressures demanding your attention, having a set organizational system can be a lifesaver, literally.

PROVIDER	PROVIDER'S NAME	CONTACT INFO	FREQUENCY	PORTAL	PORTAL PASSWORD
Primary Care					
Dentist					
Specialist 1					
Specialist 2					
Specialist 3					
Specialist 4					
Specialist 5					
Specialist 6					

James Lemons, III©

Health Screening Recommendations

To personalize your individual's healthcare screening frequency, your primary care physician is a great starting point. Your doctor may want to change monitoring frequency, or there may be some recommendations on modifications your individual needs during the test. For example, your child may need an advocate present to help calm them during the exam or to help them listen to the doctor's advice by interpreting what is said in a way your individual is more likely to understand. Your individual may need explanations about when to take medications and what their responsibilities are for their own care. It's important to have that previously identified assistance person on your individual's HIPPA forms. Otherwise, the doctor will not allow them in the exam room and no medical information can be discussed with them. A list of some health recommendations with A and B prioritization can be found at: [A and B Recommendations | United States Preventive Services Taskforce (uspreventiveservicestaskforce.org)](). For your convenience, below you'll find a brief sample table of some of the most common screenings. Work with your healthcare team to fill in the frequency recommended for your individual. Widely accepted general guidelines can be found on various national health sites. I encourage you to review these guidelines with your adult and their healthcare team to determine which screenings they feel are appropriate and their recommendations for how frequently each should be performed based on the person-centered needs of your adult who has autism. As always, it is imperative you consult with your family's care providers and perform your own due diligence in these matters. This in no way constitutes medical advice.

	Recommended frequency from the Healthcare Team
Physical Exam with CBC and BMP	
Pelvic and Breast Exams (Women)	
Mammogram (Women)	
Pap Smear (Women)	
Prostrate Exam (Males)	
PSA (Males)	
Blood Pressure	
Hearing Screening	
Depression Screening	
Lipid Panel	
Prediabetes and Diabetes Testing	
Colonoscopy	
Osteoporosis	

James Lemons, III©

Medications

Drug Name	Reason	Dosage	Time	Days	Prescribing Doctor	Doctor's Number	Pharmacy	Refill Request Number
1								
2								
3								
4								
5								
6								
7								
8								
9								
10								
11								
12								
13								
14								

James Lemons, III©

Other Skills Needed

In addition to setting up appointments to see providers and complete necessary diagnostic tests, here are some other skills your individual will need to be able either to complete autonomously or to identify someone who is going to help with these tasks.

Transportation

- If they cannot drive themselves, how do they arrange transportation when an appointment requires someone else to drive them? Ex: A colonoscopy
- What steps do they need in order to reserve time in a family member's or friend's schedule for that person to be available to provide a ride or act as an advocate to help understand instructions?
- How do they arrange for transportation through a source like Medicaid or an agency where they receive services?
- Cab or rideshare, such as Uber or Lyft?
- Can the appointment be transitioned to telehealth if there is a cost or transportation barrier? Does your individual

know how to use telehealth?

Insurance

- Is it accepted and preferred by this provider, or does another provider need to be chosen?
- Is there a renewal process or yearly enrollment? How is this done? Who can assist with this if your individual cannot do this alone?
- How are premiums met? What is their process to ensure the needed premiums are paid?

Provider Payment

- Does your child need to make payments at the time of the visit?
- If payment is made after the visit, how is this done?
- What is the process if they do not have the necessary funds for their visits or treatments? Can payments be made over time? Can they make payments in advance of the treatment? Can a treatment be performed before payments are completed? Are there resources available, like patient assistance programs, if they need help?

Medication

- Does this need separate insurance? Is that in place?
- Do they have a relationship set up with a pharmacist? (Even though many practices would like you to use their pharmacy, I recommend one pharmacy that knows your individual to avoid confusion and undesired medication interactions.)
- What if the medication is too expensive? Can the provider give them sample medication until the physician's office has worked through all the processes to obtain the authorization for insurance to cover the medication? Can they work with the provider to acquire a less expensive alternative? Is there patient assistance available to help pay for it? (Note: if a medication is a name brand, not generic, you can usually find patient assistance if you look deep enough. Although the provider may not be aware of the patient assistance, you can google the name of the prescription and find the pharmaceutical company's website. This search will

usually result in a pdf assistance form. You'll need to print the form for the provider to sign.)

- Can your individual identify side effects?
- If they have side effects, what is the process for resolving this? Your individual will need to know to call, or have their previously HIPPA-appointed person call, the provider before discontinuing medications for diabetes, high blood pressure, blood thinners, or mental health.

Activity

Our individuals with autism are outstanding at all sorts of things. Unfortunately, a large percentage of those things are sedentary activities like computer skills or video games. Combined with their favorite foods that are often anything *other* than vegetables, being overweight and/or obese are challenges that many will face. Physical activity, therefore, is absolutely an integral part of medical wellness. The lack of ability to do daily activities can thwart everyone's ability to remain independent. Being able to walk, change position, clean up your body and your living quarters, and acquire and prepare food is essential to independent living. I encourage 150 minutes of activity each week. Let's define activity: Activity is moving. It can be dancing, walking on a treadmill, jogging, playing with the dog, pacing around the room, or basically anything that requires you to move your body. If there is an activity you enjoy, then do that activity. If I tell you the best activity is swimming, but you cannot access a pool, my recommendation is worthless. Also, people are not likely to stick with an activity they don't enjoy, or at the very least, don't see the results as worth the effort. One of my sons loves his bicycle and rides it daily. We have often involved the whole family in going to the recreational center to work out using stationary bikes and treadmills. Unfortunately, it is all too easy to get off a routine of movement. If that happens, start small, but do start again.

ACTIVITY GOAL	Activity	Minutes planned
Sunday		
Monday		
Tuesday		
Wednesday		
Thursday		
Friday		
Saturday		

James Lemons, III©

The goal here is not weight-related, but rather for achieving long-term health and the ability to move well because mobility and self-sufficiency go hand-in-hand. Due to the high incidence of eating disorders in the autism community, it is critical not to overemphasize the calorie count in foods or discuss your individual's body in a way that can be interpreted as negative. I have many people on my caseload who are terrified of foods making them fat or of eating something that someone has said is bad for them. My son Jason, as I mentioned earlier, tends to weigh 130 pounds or less and is nearly six-feet-two-inches tall. When he was in his early twenties, he had not eaten one of his favorite foods at a social event or even much of anything else, at all. Still, I was not alarmed because it was a good-sized gathering with several unfamiliar people. The overwhelming number of people can be enough to disrupt his eating, but then I saw him standing in the bathroom with his shirt pulled up, looking at his stomach. Someone had commented that he shouldn't eat "that" because it will make you fat. It took me several days to work through that incident and get him to eat well again.

I have also seen a tendency for someone who is concerned about the person who has autism to hover and stare as their individual takes every bite, to make sure they are eating enough. Persons with autism have reported this to me several times. Watching every bite someone eats always seems to have the same effect on them that it would have on me and probably on you. They stop eating. To help your individual prepare for independence with a healthy mindset regarding body image, it is important to avoid creating uncomfortable eating environments.

Self-care

All of the items we have discussed in the previous chapters, including good nutrition, activity, positive self-image, and medical wellness, are important factors for maintaining emotional and mental health. Everyone needs to practice self-care and boundary-setting to support their mental and emotional well-being, but if you have a mental health diagnosis, it is especially important to maintain your medical schedule of appointments. In general, though, wellness should include fun! What do you and your individual enjoy? There are myriad possibilities for fun self-care. While I find fulfillment in sewing, writing, gardening, cooking, and reading, most activities on that list are unique to me in my house. The boys enjoy a mixture of art, video games, getting together with friends and family, cleaning, laundry, and some travel. The answer to what is likely your first question when seeing that list is *yes*, I do have one son that enjoys laundry and cleaning, but the point here is everyone is unique. Self-care should explore that uniqueness.

Just as our individuals need more practice than their peers

acquiring other skills, they also need more practice developing self-care skills. Learning to have fun and enjoy life needs to be a priority. Person-centered practices should start with a statement about what every person enjoys. If this isn't happening in your individual's life, start it. Whether working on sensory challenges, meals, self-care, or anything else, we should always build on how someone finds joy.

Chapter Ten

Stepping out into the World

The bulk of strategies for working with autism are geared toward working with children. We tend to think mostly about controlling behavior and educational plans, but to live as autonomous adults who manage their own life, our individuals need skills that will facilitate not only preserving health, but also forming meaningful connections with others in their communities while they forge their own path. Socialization with peers, family, and friends are a part of establishing those connections while experiencing that trust and joy we discussed earlier. Socialization will commonly involve opportunities to eat with others, many times in public at restaurants or fast-food establishments. Eating at a restaurant without someone to support them by ordering their food means they need to learn the skills to do it on their own. A wise Scouter once told me, don't do anything for a Scout that they can do for themselves. Following this wonderful advice, I allow, and encourage, others to use the skills they already have, and if they don't yet know how to do something, I suggest they learn it.

Ordering Food

As our boys got older, their opportunities to eat at a restaurant without us increased. This induced more than a few moments of panic when we realized someone besides us would be ordering their food, which is not easy when your child has many things on their "I won't eat that" list. While we had worked on this to a degree, it was not enough, so some intense training began. When your child eats nothing on their burger except meat, cheese, and bread, telling your friend, relative, or child's teacher they do not eat condiments, onions, pickles, lettuce, or tomatoes may not translate to "you must say the words 'plain and dry'" when ordering their burger. It is important for the individual to know how to do this on their own.

Consequently, one of the basic things I encourage families to do is to teach your child early how to order their own food. It may take longer to order meals than you'd like, but it is an important ability. Start with your child's and your favorite places to eat, figure out the exact phrasing they need to know when they order their food, and then practice. Stay close and be a backup for them, but assist only if they need help. Like everything else, this is done one level at a time, but the next steps really need to happen.

You can facilitate a child in conquering this skill by using various methods when learning to order food. A script that is either memorized, written for them to read aloud, or handed to the person taking the order is helpful. Some restaurants have picture menus to help those with disabilities. These could be used by pointing to what the individual wants. Set it up for success. Let them order a part of or their whole meal with an adult to help verify and modify their order. The steps to master this skill should progress step-by-step until they can order and pay for their meal independently. If it is a restaurant that should be tipped, teach them how to calculate that tip and how to include that or where to leave it on the table. Most restaurants now have electronic means to determine the tip, usually by clicking on the appropriate percentage, which at this writing, is commonly twenty percent; however, there are still restaurants that do not have this option and sometimes technology is not working. For those occasions, it is always a good idea to teach a backup method. If they happen to be one of those individuals that see the numbers in their head, it might be easier for them to learn to divide the bill by five and use that number for the tip, or it could be a better option to demonstrate how to calculate twenty percent on their phone.

Balancing Nutrition While Eating Out

For ordering healthy options, I encourage using food apps or nutrition information on menus. While I generally don't recommend calorie counting, I believe the calorie content provided on menus and apps can help show that many foods available at restaurants provide too many calories, some providing enough for a full day. No foods are forbidden, but a reasonable compromise might be obtaining a to-go container at the beginning of the meal, putting half in the container, then enjoying what is left. The rest of the meal can be eaten later, possibly with the addition of fruits or vegetables. I prefer to work on dividing their favorite foods into more than one meal or a meal and a snack, rather than overemphasizing eating the lower calorie option on the restaurant menu. Determining how much to order, how hungry they are, and whether to eat everything that is served can be a challenge for someone with autism. Working on good relationships with food should be a family project. It never feels fair if one person is trying to abide by different rules than others. To help your individual determine how much to order, openly discuss things like how hungry they are or whether they already have eaten a larger meal that day, so maybe they don't need to eat as much now. Will they need to eat a meal with someone later? If so, they do not want to eat so much at this meal or they won't be hungry for the later planned gathering. Have they been participating in a sporting event and consequently are hungrier than usual? There may be other questions you want to add that would be appropriate to the situation. This evaluation should be a non-judgmental, honest evaluation of how much to eat. A matter-of-fact assessment also helps teach that everyone should be their own judge of how much to order and how much to eat. Your individual will appreciate feeling like everyone else in that they have the same rights for asserting their preferences, and their choices should be accepted without comment. Using this technique at a restaurant helps teach choosing reasonable amounts of food to meet hunger needs and eating until full, but not overfull. Not everyone eats three meals daily. Moreover, some days, the nutritional load at one meal may lean more heavily than normal on certain components of the meal. It is natural that we crave certain foods and want to indulge from time to time. Unfortunately, cravings are rarely for healthy choices, but whether the food craved is a salad, a carbohydrate, or a protein, the key still comes back to balance. Is your family getting proteins every day? Do vegetables have a place on their plate most days? Have they eaten some fruit lately? At times, our individuals may naturally be hungrier due to activity, but in general, on days they eat more, consider whether it is that they are hungry or whether they eat those huge servings of food just because it is there.

Frugal Eating

Eating at a restaurant is financially expensive and usually exceeds our diet's salt and fat budget if eaten too often. Moreover, adults with autism tend to be unemployed or underemployed which for most, will translate into experiencing food insecurity at one time or the other. Maybe they will be unsure if they have enough food to eat until their next paycheck. Perhaps they will need others to help provide food for them. Some will need to use SNAP (Supplement Nutrition Assistance Program) or food pantries, so your individual might need help completing appropriate forms for that type of assistance. Whatever the case, it is essential for individuals on the spectrum to learn how to purchase and prepare food at home. Keeping in mind the fact that food pantries rarely have prepackaged or ready-to-eat meals, the more cooking skills your individual has, the better. For those with no or few cooking skills, protein shakes, microwavable chicken nuggets, and a protein or granola bar are common choices. Demonstrating how to budget for food is best done by giving your individual the budget then making a field trip to the grocery store, where they need to see how much food they can buy. Then discuss which items to reduce or increase to make the budget work. You may need to create specific budgets for each food group or meal (breakfast, lunch, dinner), and snacks to help balance both the nutrition and the financial budget.

Conquering the Grocery Store

The best time to work on this is when your individual is young by taking them with you to the grocery store. We got through these experiences by naming everything on the aisle and having them repeat it as they got restless. Richard could say hundreds of words by the time he was one year old. He had no idea what they meant, but he could say them. I am sure this added to the appearance of a language loss, which is a typical part of the autism diagnosis. In reality, he never lost the ability to say all those words, but at some point, the question changed from "how many words can he say" to "how many words does he understand?" Forty years later, I am not sure it makes any difference whether it added to an actual loss. After several years, I no longer worry about the cause and more about how we get to independence.

However, if your individual is no longer a small child who can easily be guided through the store by naming all the items on the shelf and getting that free cookie from the bakery at every visit, start by making strategic visits to the store. Have a definite goal of picking up a minimal number of items. Always start with one item and then pay for it. With adults in my current work setting, I have them do this with a friend, or I'll have someone from the clinic go with them to work through this. Eventually, we plan a menu and write a grocery list. Some have found they can do this with a list in hand, but to vary their menu, they usually need help to write a new menu and grocery list. Gaining comfort in the grocery store is a step-by-step process. A helpful piece in this process may include evaluating the store's environment. Stores that are smaller, less crowded, quieter, better organized, or have a familiar person on staff may be good places to start this journey. Intermediary steps may include ordering food from a grocery app to be delivered or picked up.

Becoming Mobile

"Transportation is always a challenge for someone with a disability." WAIT! Did I hear that right? Many years ago, I was at a new-employee training for my current employer, a behavioral health facility. When this statement was made, it was the first time it had occurred to me that getting around town might challenge our boys as they age. I seldom use absolutes because someone will prove you wrong, and in our case, this trainer was correct. Transportation has been a challenge, as there are several considerations. In the state where we live, if someone has a driver's license, you must pay for them as a driver on your car insurance. When Richard was going to college, we gave him the option of we can pay for you to get a license and get a car, or we can pay for college. We simply did not have the cash for both. He chose college.

Jason's main transportation is his bicycle, which he still rides for miles every day, just as he has since he was fourteen. So, transportation for travel within a couple of miles is not a problem for him, and on days when the weather prevents him from riding, someone from his job frequently calls and asks if he wants a ride. This is not something we arranged; it happened organically, and we are very grateful.

When the boys were old enough to qualify for Social Security and received Medicaid, this came with a medical transportation perk! We started teaching the boys how to call and arrange their own transportation if we were unavailable. Initially, this included calling family members to arrange a ride if neither of us could take them for an appointment, but soon, we found ourselves part of the sandwich generation in which we needed not only to take care of the boys' needs but also those of our aging parents. It was at this point we started teaching them to schedule rides through the Medicaid service. This has now morphed into also being able to access Uber or Lyft.

Vocational training and college on the other side of the Dallas/Fort Worth metroplex added another dimension to their training. They suddenly needed access to the commuter train and the bus and the knowledge to ride them. This was foreign territory, not only for them but for us as well, so off we went on a field trip. Richard was the first to need this transportation, so the whole family caught the train and rode the route he would need to take to get to class. Later, Jason needed to take the exact same route, plus a little further, to attend vocational training. Since Richard had traveled almost to the point where Jason would need to go, and they would be together for the trip since Richard was going to be volunteering in Jason's program, we did not do a family excursion. There was one added challenge, however, in that the commute would involve an extra bus trip, which was new to both boys. They were together, though, so we felt mostly okay about it, and they kept in contact with us by phone. They handled the whole thing well without parents tagging along. Personally, for me to do the same trip, I would need one of the boys to ride with me. They do better on public transportation than I do!

Our sons have differing comfort levels with train and bus travel. Richard takes on these journeys much like I do: Okay, here is where I am going. I get on here and ride to this point and get off. WHEW! I made it! Jason, on the other hand, has the entire city map memorized. He knows when large events are happening that might interfere with his commute and what alternate routes he might want to take. Occasionally, he decides he has not seen a particular station before and maybe today he will take a different route just to see that station. Even though they are brothers, their strengths and areas of needed growth are very different from each other.

From a parental viewpoint, sending them out to travel on their own was extremely hard. There were moments when both James and I had thoughts of bailing completely out of allowing them to take public transportation without our help. We stepped out with a little bit of faith, permitting them to venture out on their own, but the journey for them and us was not without some major bumps in the road. The very first time the boys did the last leg of the journey with that extra bus ride we had not practiced, the director of the vocational program called me after they arrived to let me know they were okay, but the bus driver had experienced a seizure during the trip and another driver had been brought in to complete the route. More frighteningly, on one of Richard's solo trips, he was robbed by someone who pressured our son not only to give him the money he had in his wallet, but to walk to the ATM to get more money.

We knew very little about safety precautions when riding public transportation, but we were fortunate enough to know someone who had worked on commuter trains for years and was willing to give us some lessons. He gave us the following rules:

- Do not sit at the entrance.
- Move as needed to sit next to someone else.
- Never open your wallet on the train.

- Do not count on security guards to see everything. That is happening. There is a lot they miss.
- Study and know your route before you go.

Putting Richard back on the train two days after he was robbed was one of the toughest things I have ever had to do, but we did it. We could have done better in teaching our boys to use transportation without us being present, but in spite of our naivete, the boys did well. If you are not well versed in how to use public transportation to get around, then I hope you find someone who will teach your individual and you the ropes.

Entering the Workforce

Our journey to bring our sons into the workforce has been a mixture of positive and negative experiences that have been both rewarding and discouraging. As with everyone, our boys' experiences have been unique. Their adventures started with the same employer in volunteer positions at Cub Scout events, then went in completely different directions. Somehow, when I was in charge of an event and needed someone to work different program areas, they were "voluntold" to do some tasks. This experience proved they could handle the responsibility and eventually worked into being hired for some paid summer camp positions. Even then, I was present at the camp and busy with my own position. Originally, they reported directly to me, but eventually that changed, and their skills and responsibilities expanded. Jason even worked one summer without me or Richard onsite.

It was during our camp experience that Jason discovered he loved doing laundry. We were part of the operation that had several themed program areas which included some costumes and, of course, those costumes needed to be washed. The program started off small, so the boys and I were able to do many of the logistical tasks without assistance. One day when I was trying to make hardtack and do laundry at the same time for a cavalry program, Jason kept interrupting me to have me move the laundry from the washer to the dryer. In a moment when I was tired, I asked if I could teach Jason to do the laundry. He was fourteen at the time. I have not done my own laundry since that day, which has now been more than twenty years. Jason's love of doing laundry, which started with his fascination with watching the washer and dryer spin, eventually led him to work at a bed and breakfast for several years.

As I mentioned when discussing the train and bus rides, at one point, Jason went to a vocational program for individuals with autism and, for a short time, Richard volunteered there, using his art skills. The skills, confidence, and independence they gained in using public transportation during this time were priceless, though the experience did not lead to employment for either one.

When Jason reached his limit for educational funding, he was without any independent activities outside our home for a while. Although he was adept at cleaning and doing laundry for us, we continued to look for an employment position for him. Jason always enjoyed the friendships he made at church, and despite the rest of the family having no interest in sports, he had become a sports fanatic with his own opinions about who would and would not win each week. One day, after he and the music director had finished their regular discussion about the upcoming week's college and professional games and who they picked to win, I asked the music director if there were any opportunities for Jason to volunteer once a week. We were not looking for a paid position, but merely a place where he might have the opportunity to socialize with others on his own. Before we pulled into our driveway, I had a text. Jason could help with some vacuuming on Thursday.

He rode his bike to church that Thursday, and all went well. He enjoyed the experience, and we were thankful for an opportunity for him to socialize and work with someone else. The next Thursday was a busy day. I had a job interview, and it was Richard's birthday, so we planned to have lunch after Jason finished volunteering. I received notice that I was being hired for the position and was filling out onboarding paperwork when Justin, our youngest, came downstairs and said, "Where is Jason? I'm hungry and it's noon. I thought we were going to lunch!"

I had him call Jason and heard him say, "What do you mean you can't go to lunch because someone quit?" At my suggestion,

Justin asked his brother to find out if he could take a lunch break. The answer was yes, so we went to pick him up. When we arrived, Jason reached for the car door and started talking. "Someone quit and I got the job!" He got all this out before he even sat down. Ten years later, he is still in the same job.

Richard's path, on the other hand, took him to college. He went first to the local junior college then moved on to the Art Institute where he completed an associate degree in graphic arts, then a bachelor's degree in media arts and animation. During that time, he had a couple of brief jobs at different fast-food restaurants, which he left for other positions. Since acquiring his degree, he has had one position using his knowledge in arts, but was laid off from that job. He currently works for a local grocery where he has worked for several years.

Challenges along the Way

I do not want to leave you, dear reader, with the impression that the pathway to getting a job for someone with autism is smooth sailing. It is not. We discussed a transitional plan when the boys were in high school during their IEP meetings; however, we truly did not know what needed to be included for it to be effective. I think you just might need a crystal ball to fully wrap your brain around exactly what you should and should not include. I encourage parents to talk to other parents to help them along this path. I want to provide you with some of my thoughts, both good and bad, about this part of our autism adventures.

- Opportunities will present themselves from unexpected places. Don't disregard an opportunity because it did not come from an expected channel. Jason's bed and breakfast job came from an in-home trainer working for the Texas Department of Rehabilitative Services (DARS) going to a conference at the BnB and talking about how Jason loved cleaning and doing laundry. The BnB owner asked him if Jason were available for hire.

- Supported employment may be possible. Through DARS, a person went with Jason to learn his job at the bed and breakfast. For weeks, she worked alongside him and made sure he knew what to do and when to do it.

- When your child becomes an adult at the age of eighteen, those providing services do not have to consult you. They may very well obtain your adult child's permission to tour places the service provider thinks would be good for them without your knowledge. For example, one of Richard's teachers thought he should consider working at a place that put straws in water bottles for about six cents each. She had him sign permission to take a tour on his eighteenth birthday.
- The post-secondary financial services your individual receives may have limits. Consider carefully where to use those allocations. Vocational training should be evaluated to determine how much debt will be incurred after the funds are depleted and what kind of success rate the program you are considering has. Funds will not be available for the next great idea. Richard incurred more educational debt than we realized he would, which resulted in our not having sufficient savings to help Jason

go to another vocational program after his financial assistance ended with the completion of his first program.

- "Person-centered" thinking still applies! We found Richard being offered a job that one of his teachers thought would be good for him, two weeks before we left to go work at camp one year.
- Know the laws that apply to any financial support your adult needs. When Jason turned twenty-one, Social Security called me to set up Medicare for him. He had reached the number of quarters he needed to apply, and I had no idea. Not all surprises turn out to be happy ones, but this one was quite a pleasant surprise.
- Boundaries are appropriate. Unless a government agency finds your individual their job, that agency does not have the right to interfere with your child's work schedule and/or evaluate the employer. You do not have to accept assistance if it is not needed.

For most parents, planning for their adult child to have adequate support either through financial aid, supported employment, or solo employment is unchartered territory! Most of us never realized we would need to take such a hands-on approach to our child finding and maintaining jobs. If you have helped your child enter the workforce, then congratulations! The majority of our individuals are not employed. If you have not reached that stage, please, do not give up. There are always possibilities.

Hope is the thing with feathers
That perches in the soul
And sings the tune without words
And never stops at all. —Emily Dickinson

Conclusion

Take Home Messages

As I finished writing the last chapter, I told my husband, "I have written the last chapter; now I need to write a conclusion." He immediately replied, "There is no conclusion; the story continues." He could not be more accurate! Every day we learn something new about autism, our young men, or both. For the most part, my motto has been we do the best we can with the information we have at the time and do not look back, but there are exceptions. If I could return to homeschool days, I would make our spelling and vocabulary words based on locations and items in the house. While I would like to tell you that I would have let what others said and did affect me less, getting to the point of ignoring or taking insensitive and upsetting comments and actions with a grain of salt is a process. Even those rough moments of our lives taught me something and, better yet, how others treated the boys when we weren't present gave me a clearer understanding of the self-care and self-protective strategies which I needed to teach them.

I hope the words in this book have brought you some validation, enjoyment, and ideas for strategies you might incorporate into your family's journey. As I think back on what I have written, the bumper sticker messages I want to drive home are:

- Set boundaries!
    - Trying to accomplish too many goals simultaneously neither breeds successful strategies nor joy and pleasure. Preserve that joy you feel when you are with your family like it is your most precious treasure because it is.
- Behavior is communication!
    - Watch your individual to see what they are doing,

not what they are not doing. The clues to finding successful strategies are in what they try to communicate to you and those around them.

- Healthy habits are your friend!
    - Repeating routines helps ingrain the process into our memories and move them from short-term to long-term memories, thus increasing the likelihood our individuals will be able to navigate. These tasks should happen without you present.
- Teach how to handle a disruption in routine.
- Teach all the necessary skills.
    - List all the skills your individual would need if you were suddenly unavailable and teach them step-by-step. Let's face it, there are always skills to be learned and improved upon, no matter your life's situation. The more your individual knows, the more likely they are to be able to handle living independently.
- A growth mindset incorporates telling the truth.

- Encouragement is essential to building confidence through truthful, but edifying, conversations about goals and the work needed to achieve those goals. Improvement is always possible, regardless of the goal.

- Potential holds no limits.
  - None of us know the limits of those we are caregivers for, whether we are talking about eating a variety of foods or their academic performance. I encourage supporting the exploration of foods, but, also, of subjects that interest them. They should always be emboldened to work towards getting as close to their goals as possible.

- Sensory issues make it difficult to determine personal needs.
  - An individual with sensory issues may not be able to distinguish between hunger, reflux, or the need to soothe themselves due to a stressful situation.

Asking if they are hungry enough to eat an apple or other piece of produce may help them determine if their need is hunger or something else.

- Limit challenges in all areas of life to one at a time.
  - It is unrealistic to believe you are going to conquer picky eating, cooking, and meal planning all at once. Pick an area to concentrate your efforts, then, as success is achieved, move on to a different challenge. If the end goal is for someone to learn to write stories, but currently they are learning to spell simple words, you would start by working on learning the correct spelling for words, then move on to writing sentences, writing paragraphs, and finally stories as each of the foundational skills are achieved.

The challenges those with autism face range from picky eating to behavioral and sensory issues, finding employment, and maintaining a job. These and many other obstacles combine to make the art of planning for balanced meals, acquiring food independently, preparing it, and even being able to enjoy the result with other people a hurdle to overcome. Yet these are all essential skills for autonomous living. Working through the challenges of autism is like preparing a recipe. The ingredients include the severity of the challenge, the determination of the family, the strategies to be used, and the support systems. Step-by-step the ingredients are combined. Sometimes the ingredients mix to create delicious results that everyone enjoys, but other times the combination produces a product that is less than appealing. I am sure all of us parents and caregivers have tried interventions that created as many pleasant as disagreeable aftermaths. Parenting someone with autism is an enormous task with many facets to conquer, but just like cooking a satisfying and enjoyable meal, with time and effort the results we will see in our individuals can enable them to reach adulthood as independent, productive individuals who bring their own flavor into their relationships and experiences.

Autism Recipe: Using Trust and Joy to Take Control of Wellness

References

American Psychiatric Association. *DSM-5 Classification*. Arlington, Va: American Psychiatric Association, 2013.

Ausderau, Karla, and Malorie Juarez. "The Impact of Autism Spectrum Disorders and Eating Challenges on Family Mealtimes." *ICAN: Infant, Child, & Adolescent Nutrition* 5, no. 5 (September 3, 2013): 315–23. https://doi.org/10.1177/1941406413502808.

"Autism and Health: A Special Report by Autism Speaks Advances in Understanding and Treating the Health Conditions That Frequently Accompany Autism," n.d. https://www.autismspeaks.org/sites/default/files/2018-09/autism-and-health-report.pdf.

Baxter, Richard, and Lauren Hughes. "Speech and Feeding Improvements in Children after Posterior Tongue-Tie Release: A Case Series." *International Journal of Clinical Pediatrics* 7, no. 3 (2018): 29–35. https://doi.org/10.14740/ijcp295w.

Berry, Rashelle C., Patricia Novak, Nicole Withrow, Brianne Schmidt, Sheah Rarback, Sharon Feucht, Kristen K. Criado, and William G. Sharp. "Nutrition Management of Gastrointestinal Symptoms in Children with Autism Spectrum Disorder: Guideline from an Expert Panel." *Journal of the Academy of Nutrition and Dietetics* 115, no. 12 (December 1, 2015): 1919–27. https://doi.org/10.1016/j.jand.2015.05.016.

Centers for Disease Control and Prevention. "Diabetes Meal Planning ☐ | Eat Well with Diabetes." Centers for Disease Control and Prevention, April 19, 2023. https://www.cdc.gov/diabetes/managing/eat-well/meal-plan-method.html.

Cermak, Sharon A., Carol Curtin, and Linda G. Bandini. "Food Selectivity and Sensory Sensitivity in Children with Autism Spectrum Disorders." *Journal of the American Dietetic Association* 110, no. 2 (February 2010): 238–46. https://doi.org/10.1016/j.jada.2009.10.032.

Conway, Catherine, Sharon Lemons, and Laura Terrazas. "Academy of Nutrition and Dietetics: Revised 2020 Standards of Practice and Standards of Professional Performance for Registered Dietitian Nutritionists (Competent, Proficient, and Expert) in Intellectual and Developmental Disabilities." *Journal of the Academy of Nutrition and Dietetics* 120, no. 12 (December 2020): 2061-2075.e57. https://doi.org/10.1016/j.jand.2020.08.094.

Coulthard, Helen, and Dipti Thakker. "Enjoyment of Tactile Play Is Associated with Lower Food Neophobia in Preschool Children." *Journal of the Academy of Nutrition and*

Dietetics 115, no. 7 (July 2015): 1134–40. https://doi.org/10.1016/j.jand.2015.02.020.

Coury, Daniel L., Paul Ashwood, Alessio Fasano, George Fuchs, Maureen Geraghty, Ajay Kaul, Gary Mawe, Paul Patterson, and Nancy E. Jones. "Gastrointestinal Conditions in Children with Autism Spectrum Disorder: Developing a Research Agenda." *Pediatrics* 130, no. Supplement 2 (November 2012): S160–68. https://doi.org/10.1542/peds.2012-0900n.

Covey, Stephen M R. *The Speed of Trust : Why Trust Is the Ultimate Determinate of Success or Failure in Your Relationships, Career and Life*. London: Simon & Schuster, 2006.

Covey, Stephen M R, and Rebecca R Merrill. *The Speed of Trust: The One Thing That Changes Everything*. New York: Free Press, 2018.

Dentist, A. Z. "High-Arched Palate - AZ Dentist." azdentist.com, May 30, 2018. http://azdentist.com/conditions/high-arched-palate.

Diabetes Food Hub. "What Is the Diabetes Plate Method?," February 2020. https://www.diabetesfoodhub.org/articles/what-is-the-diabetes-plate-method.html.

Dictionary.com. "Dictionary.com - the World's Favorite Online Dictionary!," 2018. http://www.dictionary.com.

Elbossaty, Walaa Fikry. "Vitamin D Deficiency and Autism." *Advances in Pharmacoepidemiology and Drug Safety* 06, no. 03 (2017). https://doi.org/10.4172/2167-1052.1000218.

Emerson, E. "Commentary: Childhood Exposure to Environmental Adversity and the Well-Being of People with Intellectual Disabilities." *Journal of Intellectual Disability Research* 57, no. 7 (June 8, 2012): 589–600. https://doi.org/10.1111/j.1365-2788.2012.01577.x.

Felitti, Vincent J, Robert F Anda, Dale Nordenberg, David F Williamson, Alison M Spitz, Valerie Edwards, Mary P Koss, and James S Marks. "Relationship of Childhood Abuse and Household Dysfunction to Many of the Leading Causes of Death in Adults." *American Journal of Preventive Medicine* 14, no. 4 (May 1998): 245–58. https://doi.org/10.1016/s0749-3797(98)00017-8.

Fortuna, Robert J., Laura Robinson, Tristram H. Smith, Jon Meccarello, Beth Bullen, Kathryn Nobis, and Philip W. Davidson. "Health Conditions and Functional Status in Adults with Autism: A Cross-Sectional Evaluation." *Journal of General Internal Medicine* 31, no. 1 (September 11, 2015): 77–84. https://doi.org/10.1007/s11606-015-3509-x.

Fraker, Cheri, Mark Fishbein Dr, Sibyl Cox, and Laura Walbert. *Food Chaining*. Da Capo Press, 2009.

Goday, Praveen S., Susanna Y. Huh, Alan Silverman, Colleen T. Lukens, Pamela Dodrill, Sherri S. Cohen, Amy L. Delaney, et al. "Pediatric Feeding Disorder." *Journal of Pediatric Gastroenterology and Nutrition* 68, no. 1 (January 1, 2019): 124–29. https://doi.org/10.1097/MPG.0000000000002188.

Goldschmidt, Janice, and Hee-Jung Song. "At-Risk and Underserved: A Proposed Role for Nutrition in the Adult Trajectory of Autism." *Journal of the Academy of Nutrition and Dietetics* 115, no. 7 (July 2015): 1041–47. https://doi.org/10.1016/j.jand.2015.02.013.

Goldschmidt, Janice, and Hee-Jung Song. "Development of Cooking Skills as Nutrition Intervention for Adults with Autism and Other Developmental Disabilities." *Journal of the Academy of Nutrition and Dietetics* 117, no. 5 (May 2017): 671–79. https://doi.org/10.1016/j.jand.2016.06.368.

Gray, Carol, and Jenison Public Schools (Mich. *The New Social Story Book*. Jenison, Mich.: Jenison Public Schools ; Arlington, Tx, 1998.

Groce, N., E. Challenger, R. Berman-Bieler, A. Farkas, N. Yilmaz, W. Schultink, D. Clark, C. Kaplan, and M. Kerac. "Malnutrition and Disability: Unexplored Opportunities for Collaboration." *Paediatrics and International Child Health* 34, no. 4 (October 13, 2014):

308–14. https://doi.org/10.1179/2046905514y.0000000156.

Guan, Joseph, and Guohua Li. "Injury Mortality in Individuals with Autism." *American Journal of Public Health* 107, no. 5 (May 2017): 791–93. https://doi.org/10.2105/ajph.2017.303696.

Hastings, R. P., D. Gillespie, S. Flynn, R. McNamara, Z. Taylor, R. Knight, E. Randell, et al. "Who's Challenging Who Training for Staff Empathy towards Adults with Challenging Behaviour: Cluster Randomised Controlled Trial." *Journal of Intellectual Disability Research* 62, no. 9 (July 23, 2018): 798–813. https://doi.org/10.1111/jir.12536.

Hirvikoski, Tatja, Ellenor Mittendorfer-Rutz, Marcus Boman, Henrik Larsson, Paul Lichtenstein, and Sven Bölte. "Premature Mortality in Autism Spectrum Disorder." *British Journal of Psychiatry* 208, no. 3 (March 2016): 232–38. https://doi.org/10.1192/bjp.bp.114.160192.

King, Jessica L., Jamie L. Pomeranz, and Julie W. Merten. "Nutrition Interventions for People with Disabilities: A Scoping Review." *Disability and Health Journal* 7, no. 2 (April 2014): 157–63. https://doi.org/10.1016/j.dhjo.2013.12.003.

Lai, Meng-Chuan, Caroline Kassee, Richard Besney, Sarah Bonato, Laura Hull, William Mandy, Peter Szatmari, and

Stephanie H. Ameis. "Prevalence of Co-Occurring Mental Health Diagnoses in the Autism Population: A Systematic Review and Meta-Analysis." *SSRN Electronic Journal* 6, no. 10 (2019). https://doi.org/10.2139/ssrn.3310628.

Lange, Klaus W., Joachim Hauser, and Andreas Reissmann. "Gluten-Free and Casein-Free Diets in the Therapy of Autism." *Current Opinion in Clinical Nutrition and Metabolic Care* 18, no. 6 (November 2015): 572–75. https://doi.org/10.1097/mco.0000000000000228.

Ledford, Jennifer R., and David L. Gast. "Feeding Problems in Children with Autism Spectrum Disorders." *Focus on Autism and Other Developmental Disabilities* 21, no. 3 (August 2006): 153–66. https://doi.org/10.1177/10883576060210030401.

Lefter, Radu, Alin Ciobica, Daniel Timofte, Carol Stanciu, and Anca Trifan. "A Descriptive Review on the Prevalence of Gastrointestinal Disturbances and Their Multiple Associations in Autism Spectrum Disorder." *Medicina* 56, no. 1 (December 27, 2019): 11. https://doi.org/10.3390/medicina56010011.

Lemons, Sharon. "Review of Sensory Processing Disorder, Autism and Food Challenges." *BHNewsletter* 34, no. 2 (2016): 8–10.

Lockner, Donna W., Terry K. Crowe, and Betty J. Skipper. "Dietary Intake and Parents' Perception of Mealtime Behaviors in Preschool-Age Children with Autism Spectrum Disorder and in Typically Developing Children." *Journal of the American Dietetic Association* 108, no. 8 (August 2008): 1360–63. https://doi.org/10.1016/j.jada.2008.05.003.

MA, Courtney E. Ackerman. "10 Person-Centered Therapy Techniques & Interventions [+PDF]." PositivePsychology.com, July 21, 2017. http://positivepsychology.com/client-centered-therapy/.

Mandell, David S., Christine M. Walrath, Brigitte Manteuffel, Gina Sgro, and Jennifer A. Pinto-Martin. "The Prevalence and Correlates of Abuse among Children with Autism Served in Comprehensive Community-Based Mental Health Settings." *Child Abuse & Neglect* 29, no. 12 (December 2005): 1359–72. https://doi.org/10.1016/j.chiabu.2005.06.006.

Marcason, Wendy. "What Is the Current Status of Research Concerning Use of a Gluten-Free, Casein-Free Diet for Children Diagnosed with Autism?" *Journal of the American Dietetic Association* 109, no. 3 (March 2009): 572. https://doi.org/10.1016/j.jada.2009.01.013.

Martin-Biggers, Jennifer, Kim Spaccarotella, Amanda Berhaupt-Glickstein, Nobuko Hongu, John Worobey, and Carol

Byrd-Bredbenner. "Come and Get It! A Discussion of Family Mealtime Literature and Factors Affecting Obesity Risk1–3." *Advances in Nutrition* 5, no. 3 (May 1, 2014): 235–47. https://doi.org/10.3945/an.113.005116.

mtdh.ruralinstitute.umt.edu. "Nutrition for Individuals with Intellectual or Developmental Disabilities «Montana Disability and Health Program," n.d. https://mtdh.ruralinstitute.umt.edu/?page_id=813.

"National Autism Association 2017 Impact & Advances 2017 Annual Report," n.d. https://nationalautismassociation.org/wp-content/uploads/2017/12/NAA-2017-Impact-Report.pdf.

Nugent, James T., Christine Bakhoum, Lama Ghazi, and Jason H. Greenberg. "Screening for Hypertension in Children with and without Autism Spectrum Disorder." *JAMA Network Open* 5, no. 4 (April 6, 2022): e226246–46. https://doi.org/10.1001/jamanetworkopen.2022.6246.

Park, Hye Ran, Jae Meen Lee, Hyo Eun Moon, Dong Soo Lee, Bung-Nyun Kim, Jinhyun Kim, Dong Gyu Kim, and Sun Ha Paek. "A Short Review on the Current Understanding of Autism Spectrum Disorders." *Experimental Neurobiology* 25, no. 1 (2016): 1. https://doi.org/10.5607/en.2016.25.1.1.

Peregrin, Tony. "Registered Dietitians' Insights in Treating Autistic Children." *Journal of the American Dietetic*

Association 107, no. 5 (May 2007): 727–30. https://doi.org/10.1016/j.jada.2007.03.021.

Prosser, Sarah Jean Kathryn. "Picky Eating Redefined: Exploring the Extreme Food Behaviour and Feeding Environment Challenges in Children with Autism Spectrum Disorder." ir.library.ontariotechu.ca, July 1, 2014. https://ir.library.ontariotechu.ca/handle/10155/436.

Ptomey, Lauren T., and Wendy Wittenbrook. "Position of the Academy of Nutrition and Dietetics: Nutrition Services for Individuals with Intellectual and Developmental Disabilities and Special Health Care Needs." *Journal of the Academy of Nutrition and Dietetics* 115, no. 4 (April 2015): 593–608. https://doi.org/10.1016/j.jand.2015.02.002.

Sinha, Pawan. "How Brains Learn to See." www.ted.com, February 25, 2010. http://www.ted.com/talks/pawan_sinha_how_brains_learn_to_see.

Sinha, Pawan, Margaret M. Kjelgaard, Tapan K. Gandhi, Kleovoulos Tsourides, Annie L. Cardinaux, Dimitrios Pantazis, Sidney P. Diamond, and Richard M. Held. "Autism as a Disorder of Prediction." *Proceedings of the National Academy of Sciences of the United States of America* 111, no. 42 (October 21, 2014): 15220–25. https://doi.org/10.1073/pnas.1416797111.

Smith DaWalt, Leann, Jinkuk Hong, Jan S Greenberg, and Marsha R Mailick. "Mortality in Individuals with Autism Spectrum Disorder: Predictors over a 20-Year Period." *Autism* 23, no. 7 (February 28, 2019): 1732–39. https://doi.org/10.1177/1362361319827412.

SOS Approach to Feeding. "SOS Educational Programs." Accessed November 16, 2023. https://sosapproachtofeeding.com/sos-educational-programs.

Späth, Elisabeth M. A., and Karin R. Jongsma. "Autism, Autonomy, and Authenticity." *Medicine, Health Care and Philosophy* 23, no. 1 (June 4, 2019): 73–80. https://doi.org/10.1007/s11019-019-09909-3.

Tathgur, Manmeet Kaur, and Harmeet Kaur Kang. "Challenges of the Caregivers in Managing a Child with Autism Spectrum Disorder— a Qualitative Analysis." *Indian Journal of Psychological Medicine* 43, no. 5 (April 12, 2021): 025371762110007. https://doi.org/10.1177/02537176211000769.

Walker, Harry A. "Incidence of Minor Physical Anomaly in Autism." *Journal of Autism and Childhood Schizophrenia* 7, no. 2 (June 1977): 165–76. https://doi.org/10.1007/bf01537727.

Weise, Janelle, Karen R Fisher, Erin Whittle, and Julian N Trollor. "What Can the Experiences of People with an

Intellectual Disability Tell Us about the Desirable Attributes of a Mental Health Professional?" *Journal of Mental Health Research in Intellectual Disabilities* 11, no. 3 (May 17, 2018): 183–202. https://doi.org/10.1080/19315864.2018.1469700.

Wigham, Sarah, Chris Hatton, and John L. Taylor. "The Effects of Traumatizing Life Events on People with Intellectual Disabilities: A Systematic Review." *Journal of Mental Health Research in Intellectual Disabilities* 4, no. 1 (March 4, 2011): 19–39. https://doi.org/10.1080/19315864.2010.534576.

www.unicef.org. "The State of the World's Children 2013," n.d. https://www.unicef.org/reports/state-worlds-children-2013.

Appendix
Menu Planning Sheet

Menu

Entrée:
Ingredients needed:
1. _____
2. _____
3. _____
4. _____
5. _____
6. _____

Entrée Cooking Instructions

Time to prepare entree recipe:
Start preparing at:

Starch:
Ingredients needed:
1. _____
2. _____
3. _____
4. _____
5. _____
6. _____

Starch Cooking Instructions

Time to prepare starch recipe:
Start preparing at:

Vegetable:
Ingredients needed:
1. _____
2. _____
3. _____
4. _____
5. _____
6. _____

Vegetable Cooking Instructions

Time to prepare vegetable recipe:
Start preparing at:

James Lemons, III©

Lemons' Food Project Examples

For each food, we tried four different recipes that allowed us to try different textures and flavors while we also incorporating some elements that were already accepted by most, if not all, of us when possible. Below you'll find some examples and ideas

Green beans:

Green Beans with potatoes, bacon, garlic, and small potato pieces

Air fried green beans with garlic powder and salt

Pan braised green beans with lemon and onion powder

Oven roasted green beans with lemon and garlic

Oranges:

Peeled fresh oranges

Fruit cup oranges

Orange juice

Orange chicken

Lemons:

Girl Scout lemon cookies

Lemon garlic chicken

Oven roasted potatoes with lemon and dill

Lemon cream pie

Sweet Potatoes:

Sweet potato hash

Baked sweet potatoes

Sweet potato fries

Baked sweet potatoes

Cranberries: (We have tried these several ways for Thanksgiving, mainly cooked on the stovetop.)

Cranberries with sugar and water – no extra flavor

Cranberries with lemon zest, sugar, and water

Cranberries with vanilla, sugar, water, and orange zest

Cranberries with maple flavoring, sugar, water, and lemon juice

Future plans include cranberry bread, cranberry pancakes, cranberry salad.

Recipe Modifications
Or Rewriting a Recipe to Fit the Need

Equipment and Utensils: I start with equipment and utensils because many individuals with autism are afraid of these. It really does not matter how the fear originated, but if fear exists, it will be a barrier to learning cooking skills. Look at what is needed to complete a recipe. Could less fear-inducing alternatives be used? Some introductory equipment that could be considered are crock pots or electric skillets instead of stoves. A plastic lettuce knife helps if cutting is involved, as long as you do not really need a sharp knife to complete the tasks. Modifying equipment will also allow you to move the setting to a room outside of the kitchen. Many times, the fear might be the location, itself. As always, take precautions for safety, but remember some of the fear our individuals experience is because of something that was *said* in the past, rather than the actual act of cooking or using utensils.

Ingredients: Especially when first starting to cook, it is a good idea to look for ingredients that do not need as much preparation.

You may find incorporating precooked chicken makes the recipe a success, but cooking raw chicken might be too much of a stretch due to sensory challenges, anxiety over spending too much time in the kitchen, or fears of making someone else sick because the meat was not cooked long enough. There are many alternatives to ingredients. Consider an onion. You can buy it minced, powdered, chopped, dried, or chopped and frozen. Other options are onions that are easier to slice like a green onion, or changes in the instructions, like using a chopper to cut it. I use the search engine on my favorite grocery app to get ideas on what food ingredients I can change to make the process less intimidating or to shorten the time needed to prepare ingredients.

Adding pictures: As mentioned previously, having pictures of the exact ingredients and utensils can be very beneficial. It can also be helpful to have a picture of your cooking timer with the correct time or your cooking thermometer with the correct internal temperature, especially in the beginning. As with other skills, a good goal is to work towards being able to use something similar, but not exactly like the picture. As we already discussed, food companies change their labels, and utensils like measuring cups can be lost or come to an unfortunate end, like when one of the boys left my Tupperware measuring cup in the dog food. When the dog got into the bag of food, my measuring cup was destroyed.

Short Precise Instructions: Wordy recipe instructions can be confusing. One of the most important steps is to remove any confusing instructions. I have found recipes from food companies to be particularly troublesome as they tend to include practically a complete advertising campaign in the list. If I can get away with three of four words, that is great! Sometimes, it takes more, but limit the words to as few as possible.

Make it a Family Project: The first time you try a modified recipe, you will almost always find there are still changes to be made. The exact time it takes to cook a chicken dish using pre-cooked chicken instead of raw chicken will differ, for example. Make the recipe with your individual and adjust the recipe to be more precise for the next time.

Autism Recipe: Using Trust and Joy to Take Control of Wellness

Recipe

Ingredients

1 _____

2 _____

3 _____

4 _____

5 _____

Time to prepare:

Time to cook:

James Lemons, III©

Recipe

Instructions

1 ———————

2 ———————

3 ———————

4 ———————

5 ———————

Time to prepare:
Time to cook:

Sample Doctor's Letter

Date

Dear [Insert Physician's Name]:

My name is [Insert Individual's Name]. I have a diagnosis of Autism Spectrum Disorder. I wanted to provide you with some information to help you give me better medical care.

Some accommodations I may need when being examined are: [Insert needs. Possible needs include: someone on the HIPAA list present (list exact names), extra time for instructions, frequent checks for understanding, instructions that are written, a male or female present, providing numbers when requesting I call someone else for further care, time spent talking to me about my favorite things to help reduce my anxiety, short waits in the lobby, and any others that you, as caregiver, feel are needed.]

The person/people authorized to assist me with medical decisions is/are: [Insert name]. I will provide documentation.

My current medical diagnoses are: [Insert medical diagnoses]

My current behavioral diagnoses are: [Insert behavioral diagnosis]

Medications I take are: [Insert medications]

My activity routine: [Insert routine]

Some of my favorite things: [Insert top 5 list]

Things that are important to me [Insert top 5 list]

Sincerely,

Individual's Name

www.ingramcontent.com/pod-product-compliance
Lightning Source LLC
Chambersburg PA
CBHW070528090426
42735CB00013B/2909